Pilates *lite*

Pilates *lite*

EASY EXERCISES TO LOSE WEIGHT AND TONE UP

KARON KARTER

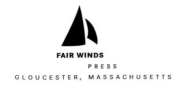

FAIR WINDS
PRESS
GLOUCESTER, MASSACHUSETTS

First published in the USA in 2004 by
Fair Winds Press
33 Commercial Street
Gloucester, MA 01930

08 07 06 05 04   1 2 3 4 5

ISBN 1-59233-083-5

Library of Congress Cataloging-in-Publication Data available

Cover design by Mary Ann Smith
Book design by Yee Design

Printed and bound in Singapore

The information in this book is for educational purposes only. It is not intended to replace the advice of a physician or medical practitioner. Please see your health care provider before beginning any new health program.

To Gilda's Girls

CONTENTS

6

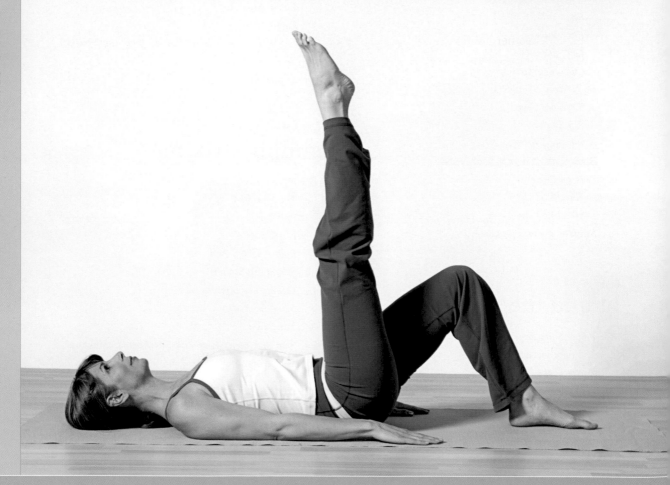

INTRODUCTION

WOULDN'T YOU LOVE TO CHANGE YOUR BODY?
Those of us who do Pilates know that you can—not in an invasive,
harsh way that stresses your body, but in a subtle way that results
in permanent changes. You will have long and strong muscles, a
firm and flat tummy, and a taller and tighter appearance! Your
posture will improve and you will feel revitalized. Maybe this
sounds great and you would love to try Pilates, but feel it's too difficult. My own mother felt that regular Pilates classes were too
hard. She is a healthy woman despite never having stepped a foot
inside a gym—she hates to exercise, but expressed an interest in
learning Pilates. I was thrilled to introduce her to Pilates, but
found my teaching skills challenged. She couldn't do many of the
exercises. And honestly, many of my students can't! You need a
fair amount of abdominal strength going into a Pilates class in
order to do the exercises correctly; otherwise, you risk straining or
injuring yourself. My fear was that the usual exercises and their
many directions would be overwhelming and turn her off to
Pilates forever. Enter *Pilates Lite*!

As a direct result of these experiences, the approach I take in
Pilates Lite begins long before the first exercise. Because Pilates
retrains your body's movements, much of what you'll do is based
on progression. *Pilates Lite* will prepare your body so that you can
work safely (and sanely) without straining yourself in the process.
By following the techniques presented in this book, I hope that
you'll be ready to walk into a Pilates mat class feeling confident
and secure.

Chapter 1, "The Pilates Lite Body," will explain what this book can offer you. I have seen my students' bodies change, especially their waists, but that is just one of many benefits. You, too, will come to understand what makes Pilates so special. It is built on a solid foundation that you can trust to bring you greater health and self-confidence.

In chapter 2, "Fusing Mind and Motion," you'll come to understand why this method works. Pilates is founded on six guiding principles, and because this 90-year-old method is so sound, it has introduced the importance of core strength to practitioners throughout the world.

We all want to grow and be inspired. Chapter 3, "Soothe and Move," introduces you to a body journey that will move you to excel. A series of awareness exercises will show you how to move your body toward health and fitness. This will be your first attempt to retrain your body's movements, muscle by muscle, and to come to understand your own body's complexities.

With a comprehensive understanding of your body's limitations and strengths, you can advance to chapter 4, "Fit and Lite." In this chapter, you'll begin to build overall body strength, integrate your mind and muscles, and strengthen the muscles that stabilize and support your spine.

In chapter 5, "One Muscle at a Time," you'll gain more strength, coordination, and balance—all ingredients of functional fitness—to get your body ready for whatever life throws your way. These exercises prepare you for your own beginner mat class in chapter 6, "Simply Striking." In this chapter, you'll enjoy moving through the ten exercises that make up a classic beginner Pilates mat class. These exercises, along with the leg series, are guaranteed to tighten and tone key areas throughout your body. This is the real deal! Soon you'll experience the magic of Pilates. I hope you come to love it as much as I do!

THE PILATES LITE SOLUTION

———————— ✳ ————————

Sometimes, it takes a total stranger to make you stop and think. I had such a moment about two years ago when I walked into a classroom ready and excited to teach Pilates to the women of Gilda's Club of North Texas. These women were a blessing and an inspiration; they stretched me to my limits—to be a better teacher! I knew in advance that I would be teaching women living with cancer, but I was not really prepared. Since they showed no visible signs of their illness, I figured that a modified Pilates class would be fine. Well, I was wrong. Many of the exercises were too difficult for them. They didn't seem to mind, but I did. I was not comfortable putting them in a situation where they would question their bodies. After all, they needed to heal, emotionally and physically. For the first time, I was intellectually challenged by how to teach Pilates. So, I asked myself: How do I build body awareness while balancing their physical and emotional needs? How can I teach them within an hour-long class to safely move their bodies, knowing that even the slightest movement could help them heal? How can I strengthen their bodies to prepare them for a traditional Pilates mat class?

As those questions played out in my head, I tried various exercises and found I always came back to the fundamentals of Pilates. As I experimented, my students thrived. And that's how I came up with Pilates Lite.

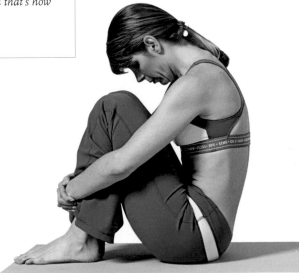

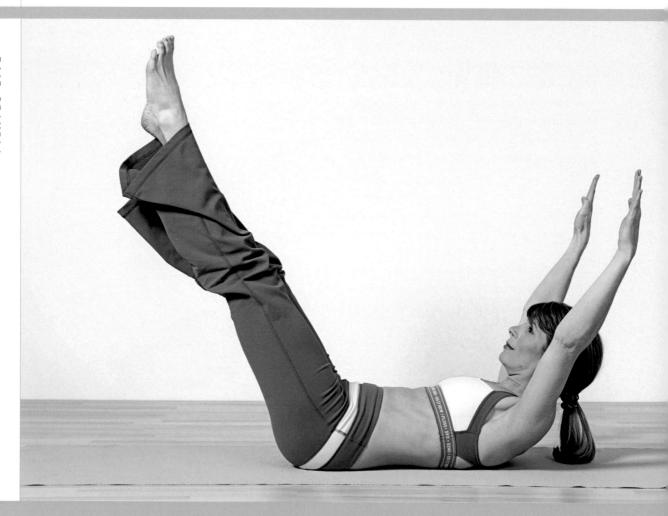

THE PILATES LITE BODY

IN A PERFECT WORLD, we would all have amazing abs and no love handles around the waist. But we don't live in a perfect world, which leaves us searching for effective ways to trim and tone our tummies. Many of the exercise programs that promise to strengthen and trim torsos also put a lot of stress on the body. So I wondered, can I create a gentler approach to fitness that can give my students their best bodies—and abs to envy? Introducing Pilates Lite!

While strict Pilates is a vigorous fitness method, Pilates Lite presents a much more subtle approach to the exercises. These gentle movements will give you all the benefits of Pilates, such as the long and strong muscles of a ballerina, a firm and flat tummy, and a taller and toned appearance— not to mention a tighter tush! But that's not all. Each exercise emphasizes correct alignment, so that as the muscles that support your spine get stronger, your posture will improve—and you will feel revitalized. With Pilates Lite, not only will you enjoy the stretching benefits of yoga, but you

THE PILATES PROMISE

✳

Pilates is a fitness regime that uses equipment for resistance as well as a series of floor exercises to tone your body, increase flexibility, improve your balance and coordination, and create a fusion between your mind and body.

will also build strength without adding muscle bulk. Pilates exercises focus on the development of muscular harmony and balance, not just size. Pilates Lite still strengthens the key muscles in your body, only more gently than a traditional Pilates workout. In other words, the essence of Pilates is still very much alive in my program, only the physical movements are modified to make them easier and more accessible.

Imported Fitness: Joseph Pilates

To understand Pilates origin, let's travel back to the birth of Joseph Hubertus Pilates. He was born near Dusseldorf in Germany in 1880. As a child, he was frail and prone to diseases, such as asthma, rickets, and rheumatic fever. Intrigued by physical fitness and driven because of his own childhood diseases, he studied both Eastern and Western forms of exercise. Everything from yoga, Zen, and ancient Greek and Roman regimens to studying animal movements gave him ideas for his fitness method. To improve his own wellbeing, he worked everyday to build his body toward better health. His love of and interest in physical fitness led him to explore various sports. He eventually became an accomplished athlete, mastering sports such as diving, skiing, boxing, and gymnastics.

In 1912, Pilates left his native Germany for England to pursue a career in boxing. But his career was cut short as a result of World War I, when the British authorities detained him as a German National. For the next twelve months, he taught his fellow prisoners of war his version of the ideal physical fitness regimen. He was confident that they would emerge stronger than they were before their confinement—and they did. Legend has it that none of his followers fell ill to the influenza epidemic that swept the nation and killed thousands of people. Interestingly, those same exercises are taught today—and you'll see them in this book.

While in camp, Pilates garnered the reputation of a legendary healer. As the men were convalescing from wartime diseases, he invented new ways to help rehabilitate them. If individuals, for example, were bedridden, he attached springs to their beds, to get them moving. Perhaps he instinctively knew new that any movement is better than no movement, and that any movement

THE IDEAL FITNESS

———— ✳ ————

Joseph Pilates wrote in 1945: "The definition of the ideal physical fitness: The attainment and maintenance of a uniformly developed body with a sound mind fully capable of naturally, easily and satisfactorily performing our many and varied daily tasks with spontaneous zest and pleasure."

would increase their body's circulation and therefore they would heal better.

After the war, Joseph Pilates returned to Germany to continue his work. Because he was so successful at healing and training, he caught the eye of the dance world, and many dancers and athletes turned to him for physical training—it is interesting to think that he may have been the world's first personal (physical) trainer. During that time, his methods caught the attention of the New German Army, but he decided against teaching them. Soon he left for America.

As he crossed the Atlantic, Pilates met his future wife, Clara, a nurse. Together, they opened a studio in the same New York City building that held the New York City Ballet. Pilates was not an instant success, however. Eventually his ideal fitness caught the attention of the ballet community, including elite dancers, such as Martha Graham and George Balanchine. Dancers, because of their grueling physical schedules, are prone to injuries, and as word spread that Joseph Pilates' method reduced recovery time, they flocked to his studio. His teachings became (and still are) an integral part of the dance community. In fact, if not for a handful of his most devoted and faithful students (most of them dancers), his teachings might not be as popular today. Much of what is taught in today's studios has been passed down through generations of teachers, spreading his methods worldwide. And although Joseph Pilates' essential message is ninety years old, it still continues to deliver results!

Why Pilates Lite?

Pilates, like any form of movement, can lead to injury when performed incorrectly. *Pilates Lite,* however, will provide basic fundamentals so you can practice safely and correctly. Over many years as a teacher, I have found that no two people are alike, whether healthy or health-challenged. Some of my students cannot touch their toes while others have Gumbi-like flexibility. Remarkably, a few of my seriously health-challenged students run triathlons, whereas many of my healthy students choose not to. Of course, I believe Pilates exercises are life transforming, but I am the first to recognize that some of the exercises are physically challenging,

WORDS FROM
JOSEPH PILATES:
THE PROPHECY

*"In 10 sessions, you will
feel the difference;
in 20, you will see the difference;
and in 30, you will have
a whole new body."*

which is why I created this book—to prepare your body for this transformation.

My goals are to give you all that Pilates embodies—its techniques and principles. Most importantly, I hope to teach you how to exercise with good alignment and empower you to get to know yourself so you can make an informed decision on what is right for your body—particularly what exercises are appropriate for you. In general, proper alignment means that you are able to hold your entire body and all its individual parts in their place so that they can perform with maximum economy of movement and minimum wear on your body. Developing your inner consciousness will help protect you from injuries on and off the mat, which is the best gift you can give yourself.

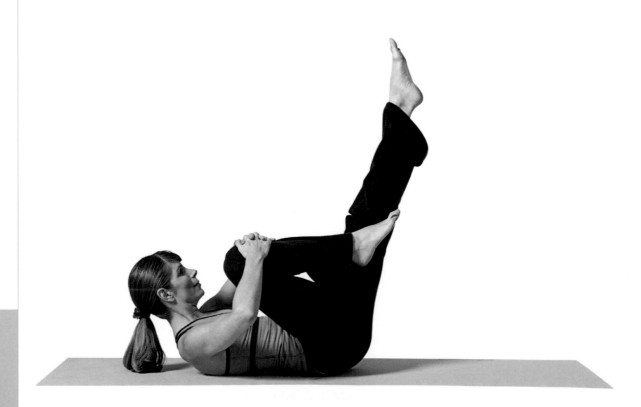

Pilates Lite is the right program for you if:

* You think a traditional Pilates mat class is too difficult for you to start with.

* You are intimidated by group exercise settings.

* You are starting an exercise program for the first time or you are getting back into shape after pregnancy or injury.

* You suffered a minor injury and cannot do your normal fitness workout, yet want to stay conditioned.

* You find that what you used to do for fitness may not be so good for your body now.

* You are interested in easing some of the symptoms of chronic illnesses, such as osteoporosis and arthritis.

* Your back is chronically tender and sore, and you are searching for pain relief.

* Your doctor or physical therapists suggested Pilates and yet you feel uncomfortable trying to learn a whole new exercise routine, especially if you are under a great deal of stress.

* You are ready to diminish those love handles around your waist—in this case, it's okay to be love*less*!

More than a Method

I am inviting you to try *Pilates Lite* right now. Your age, physical limitations, or athletic abilities do not matter. Pilates works for many different types of people, so anyone can benefit from the gentle exercises and techniques presented in this book. The aim is not to sweat it out or build muscle bulk as you count rep after rep, but rather to perform the movement correctly and mindfully (which is why some exercises are more gentle and are done at a slower pace with fewer repetitions). You will use various props, such as a pillow off your bed (nothing fancy), to ensure proper body alignment. Quality over quantity always prevails.

These workouts are goal oriented. Each chapter increases in intensity so you can build strength and confidence while gaining flexibility and knowledge. My ultimate goal (and there is no time limit on this) is for you to be able to perform the traditional Pilates mat class presented at the end of this book—if you so choose. In honoring the spirit of Pilates, the exercises in this book are bio-mechanically safe and non-impact oriented. Each exercise focuses on stretching and strengthening all the major muscle groups in your body without neglecting the smaller ones. You can do these exercises in the privacy and comfort of your own living room, or take this book with you while traveling.

Pilates Lite can be your primary mode of body conditioning and injury prevention, or you can supplement it with your own weekly exercise routine. If this is your first attempt at fitness, please follow the beginner workout for at least six weeks and try to do the routine three to four times a week. Keep in mind, these exercises are not just exercises; *Pilates Lite* is a path to lifelong fitness and mindful health. Benefits include:

* STRENGTHENING YOUR POWERHOUSE. Besides a firmer and flatter torso, you will strengthen your *powerhouse*. Joseph Pilates coined this term, meaning a central girdle of strength which includes the muscles of your abdominals, back, hips, and buttocks. Every movement in life, whether sitting or walking, requires strength from your powerhouse, which is why virtually all the exercises in this book strengthen this area. Your abs, hips, and lower back will ultimately develop into a strong support center for your everyday activities. Your core is your body's source of power!

* COORDINATING YOUR MIND AND BODY. In the early stages, Joseph Pilates called his method Contrology. In his original book, *Return to Life Through Contrology*, Pilates wrote, "Ideally, our muscles should obey our will, reasonably, our will should not be dominated by the reflex actions of our muscles." In other words, your mind will tell your body what it needs. No motion will happen without thinking about it first. Pilates is a well organized fitness program designed to work various muscle groups at the same time, creating an internal process that will align your body and change your life. With this heightened level of mind and body integration, you can exercise safely and have complete control over your body.

* IMPROVING YOUR BALANCE. Balance plays a vital role in your daily life and yet you may take it for granted. However, with age, your balance skills will quickly diminish. The exercises in this book will not only help you strengthen the muscles of your core—a vital component of balance—but you will do these exercises on the floor in a variety of positions, strengthening the muscles of your feet, ankles, and legs, which keep you standing upright in the first place.

PILATES FOR HIRE

*

If you decide that you need some hands-on guidance with this book, think about hiring a private instructor. You can tailor your private sessions to your specific needs with either a mat class or with a variety of machines, such as the Universal Reformer, the Cadillac, the Wunda Chair, and the Barrels. Besides having lots of fun, you get the individual attention from an instructor who can correct your movements, fine-tune your body alignment, and make you more confident in your own abilities when you decide to work on the exercises at home.

✳ ELIMINATING MUSCULAR IMBALANCES. Life has a way of making you a little off balance, whether in your body or life in general. Gravity makes your body droop and everyday habits can alter your appearance and posture. Slumping around your office can round your shoulders, eventually making you a few inches shorter. Playing sports that use only one side of your body will make that side stronger. While having a career and a healthy lifestyle are important, repeatedly overusing certain parts of your body can be detrimental, unless you have a way to counterbalance such behavior. The exercises in this book will help correct muscular imbalances by first drawing your attention to such issues, and then by realigning your body, muscle by muscle, to help offset existing imbalances and keep you from developing new ones.

✳ LENGTHENING YOUR LOOK. The hallmark of Pilates is that it lengthens your body and gives you a dancer's strong, lean, flexible physique. Length in a muscle means more strength as well—as you develop more muscle fibers within the muscle itself, it will get stronger. Wouldn't you love to have the tremendous strength of ballerinas—and wouldn't we all love to have their bodies?

PILATES AND PREGNANCY

———— ✳ ————

Should you do Pilates when you are pregnant? The answer depends on whether or not you were doing Pilates beforehand. If not, then it isn't wise to begin Pilates at this time. First, the inner abdominal pull which is required in every exercise—navel to spine—may not be healthy for a new fetus. Second, Pilates can be a challenging method to learn. Why add more stress to your already stressed body by learning a new system? Of course, that decision is between you and your doctor. However, Pilates Lite is an excellent option for after your baby is born. Doing some of the pelvic floor work in this book, which is a form of Kegel, can be an excellent option for strengthening the muscles of the vagina. And the abdominal work will help you get your belly and body back into shape!

✳ STRETCHING YOUR MUSCLES. With every exercise, you will rhythmically stretch your body to improve its range of motion. Lack of flexibility often leads to aches and pains. Your body is a closed system, meaning that what happens in one part will eventually affect another part. Keeping your muscles flexible is one effective way to prevent injury. Because Pilates exercises are multi-muscle integrated, they strengthen one part of your body while lengthening another part. As a result, your overall flexibility will improve and optimal muscle length will also help your joints maintain their natural range of motion. Stretching tight muscles will help you surrender to that oh-so-delicious feeling of relaxation.

✳ DEVELOPING YOUR BREATH. Your breath fuels your body. Joseph Pilates knew this, which is why every Pilates exercise coordinates movement with breath—inhaling and exhaling at the appropriate times.

✳ RELIEVING MINOR BACK PAIN. Another hallmark of Pilates is that it can reduce most minor lower back pain because it is based on postural awareness and core training. Pilates is well accepted among the rehabilitative community, including physical therapists, chiropractors, and orthopedic surgeons, because it relieves minor back issues.

Aging Well: Invest in your Future

There are two kinds of age: your chronological age and your "real" age. You do not have to succumb to gradual physical decline just because you are adding years to your driver's license. In fact, you can grow younger everyday from this point on just by moving your body!

Nothing in life is constant, not even your body. After all, just as you can recover from an emotional problem or trauma, your body can repair damaged tissue after suffering from a devastating disease. So do not worry if you have been slow to get off the couch. You have the power within to get better each day of your life—and there is plenty of good research out there to prove it. You can take little steps everyday towards feeling great and enhancing your health. You do not have to stay the same person you were yesterday.

Exercise is your winning lottery ticket to turning back the years on your biological clock. Of course, eating well and taking time for yourself also play a major roll in how well you age, but you can start here and now with *Pilates Lite*. Rest assured, I created this book so that my own mother and anyone else could perform these exercises, regardless of age or physical abilities.

AGING AMERICA

❋

The good news is you are not aging alone! America as a whole is aging, and rapidly. By the year 2030, the aging population will grow to over 70 million. The most rapid increase of the 65-plus population will occur between 2010 and 2030. Every 7.6 seconds someone will celebrate his or her 50th birthday!

The steps you take now, no matter how small, will influence the way you feel now and later in life. As you get older, what you did yesterday may not necessarily work for you today. But you must keep moving, recognizing that exercise can help slow down your:

* Decline in muscular strength—an active person loses .5 percent of physiological strength per year; as compared to an inactive or unfit person, who loses 2 percent

* Decline in muscular power and endurance

* Decline in muscle mass—approximately 6 percent per decade after age 50

* Decline in bone mineral and density—usually 10–20 percent for women by age 65

* Decline in resting metabolism

* Decline in balance

* Decline in joint mobility

* Decline in neural or brain cells

* Decline in immunity.

* Increase in total body fat

Searching for an appropriate fitness program to meet maturing needs can be daunting. But because the exercises in this book focus on spinal alignment while strengthening the muscles that support your trunk—all vital components to aging safely—you can feel at ease about adding up the biological years. After all, your "real" age is yet to be determined! Here's what you have to look forward to with Pilates Lite:

* Increased total body strength

* Increased core strength

* Improved posture

* Lengthened body (I like to say long and luscious)

* Increased breathing capacity

* Increased flexibility

* Enhanced bone health

* Increased circulation

* Improved joint mobility

* Toned thighs and buttocks

* Heightened energy levels

* Slimmer waistline

* Fewer back aches

* Increased self confidence

Mending with the Mat

I wish I had a penny for every student that has come to me and said, "My doctor said Pilates would be good for my back injury." Well, it would be! But walking into a mat class, without knowing the fundamentals of Pilates or having developed your inner body awareness, could actually hurt your back. Not because of the teacher's inability (most Pilates instructors have a good working knowledge of how to strengthen and protect your back), but because she cannot give you the individual attention you need when she has a classroom full of students. You need to learn how to safely perform the exercises to properly recover.

Pilates Lite can be used to condition and recondition your body, so you can move through life with strength, grace, and ease of motion, ready for whatever life throws your way. However, *Pilates Lite* is not a one-time-fix-it method. You must practice and keep at it, but the payoff is huge: You will strengthen your core, which will support you entire back; you will learn how to drop your shoulders to ease chronic pain caused by upper back tension. Best of all, you will move safely in your body because *Pilates Lite* teaches you to do so.

Keep in mind that Joseph Pilates developed a system of fitness for a healthy body. He helped rehabilitate many dancers before physical therapy was a formal science, but he did this in personalized one-on-one sessions. If you are nursing a serious injury, please consult your doctor or qualified specialist before beginning this program, or you risk unconsciously overcompensating by displacing your body weight on an uninjured part of your body. This chain reaction will physically set you back even further, perhaps increasing your healing time. And if you don't perform as well as you would like, you may experience feelings of inadequacy, which might set you back emotionally as well. Don't let this happen—use the time to heal your body, not tear it down.

Although the exercises in this book are specifically modified so as not to stress your body, you may flourish under the guidance of an experienced instructor. So, what qualifications should you look for in an instructor? That is a difficult question to answer because many fine instructors complete rigorous certification programs, but do not necessarily have years of experience behind them. Look for an instructor who has been teaching for at least three to five years and is certified (preferably not only by a weekend certification program). This way, she has probably worked with a variety of bodies and can draw from her experiences.

You may also want to drop into a studio to see what is going on. Ask yourself, "Will I feel comfortable working with that person?" Many teachers are former dancers and have used some form of Pilates to heal their own bodies. Talk to your potential instructor. Another option is to find a physical therapist certified in Pilates. Because of her knowledge of anatomy, she may be an excellent person to help you with an injury. You might also want to look for an instructor specializing in re-conditioning—look for words like *Pilates-Based, Re-Conditioning,* or *Corrective Programs.* In the end, your comfort level and the trust the two of your build will move you closer to healing.

✳

Many fitness professionals advocate the stock market approach to getting healthy, meaning that to increase the rate of return on your investment—which is your body—you need to start saving now. It's never too late to start, but the younger you are, the bigger the bank account. These chapter highlights show you how *Pilates Lite* is one of the best investments you can make in your body:

* * *

Pilates Lite is based on the fundamentals of Pilates—and will prepare you for a mat class if you choose that path.

* * *

With every exercise in this book, you will gain flexibility, strength, balance, and coordination while focusing on spinal alignment.

* * *

Pilates Lite is a gentler approach to fitness. Regardless of your age, physical limitation, health, or athletic abilities, you can benefit from the techniques in this book.

* * *

Words from Joseph Pilates:
"In 10 sessions, you will feel the difference;
in 20, you will see the difference;
and in 30, you will have a whole new body."

* * *

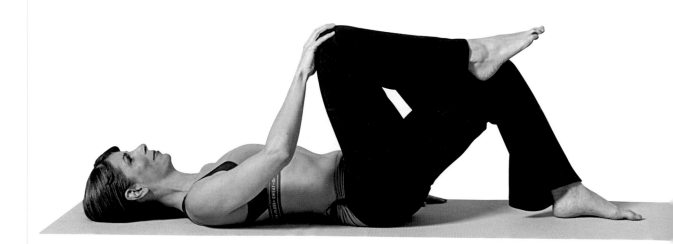

CHAPTER TWO

FUSING MIND AND MOTION

IT'S NOT WHAT YOU DO, but how you do it! Sure, you can just "make it" to exercise class. But is that all you desire? Pilates will restore healthy movement, and also align your thoughts with your body—engaging you, and cultivating a thinking body. Rather than performing mind-numbing movements, you will slow down and take the time to think about why you are doing a particular exercise. The ultimate goal, besides tightening and toning, is fusing your mind and body so that your movements come naturally with ease and proper alignment. The goal is not to wear out your body, but to inspire you to do more for yourself.

These life transforming exercises are based on six guiding principles. This chapter provides a working knowledge of these principles, allowing you to engage your brain and your body together harmoniously. You will continuously monitor your body while doing these exercises, making a mental checklist of how your body feels. Because there is no mind and body separation, this method is holistic, offering you a deeper unity of body, mind, and spirit.

The Six Guiding Principles

Joseph Pilates studied both Eastern philosophies and Western techniques to develop a hybrid exercise method. Pilates is based on six guiding principles that form its foundation. What is interesting is that these principles are simple and sound guidelines for life, not just the hour that you exercise. The six guiding principles of Pilates are:

* Concentration

* Control

* Centering

* Flow

* Precision

* Breathing

GUIDING PRINCIPLE ONE: CONCENTRATION

Before every Pilates Lite class, I ask my students to take a moment to breathe and listen to their bodies. Are they feeling tension? What can they do to be calmer? Are they stressed? With this information, they can better gauge their workout and then concentrate on their bodies. Concentration is the first guiding principle of Pilates and is so vital because it teaches you to respect every detail of your body. I also suggest that my students give themselves body reviews during the workout. Your questions may sound like this: Where is the placement of my head? Is my lower back pressed into the floor? Am I breathing or holding my breath? As minor as these details may seem, they dramatically affect the quality of the exercise. In Pilates, body positioning is the first exercise.

Start by paying attention to your body so you can become more familiar with what feels "right" and what doesn't. Joseph Pilates said, "Concentrate on the correct movements each time you exercise, lest you do them improperly and thus lose all the vital benefits of their value."

GUIDING PRINCIPLE TWO: CONTROL

Joseph Pilates designed each exercise to engage multiple muscle groups in a very precise and focused way, so you do not need to perform endless repetitions or spend hours working out. A few thoughtful exercises are far better than moving on autopilot! In addition, like concentration, control is another safety measure. I often say to my students, "No jerks in class," meaning work with control rather than jerk through the motion just to accomplish an exercise. There is no shame in admitting that an exercise is too difficult—it's so much better to modify the exercise than to struggle and use poor form. Pilates exercises are physically challenging and remembering all of the directions along with proper alignment can be draining. However, it is important to recognize that moving haphazardly through an exercise may cause you injury. Engaging your core muscles and paying close attention to body position will give you control over the exercise, allowing you to perform it correctly and safely. If you simply lack the physical strength at this time in your practice to perform an exercise with control, do not judge yourself, or feel discouraged. Accept your limitations and aim to improve from that point on.

GUIDING PRINCIPLE THREE: CENTERING

Your center is often neglected and therefore weak, which can put tremendous strain on your back. So, where is your center? Imagine a thick rubber band tightening around your middle, wrapping like a corset around your waist from below the bottom of your rib cage to your hip bones and continuing around your back ribs. This imaginary rubber band consists of many different muscles in your stomach, buttocks, hips, and back.

Centering involves correctly engaging the muscles throughout your center to protect your back and give you the proper base for all your movements; it is the focal point of Pilates. A strong center is your body's source of power. With a strong center you can lift more and run longer. Your spine can reach, lengthen, and move through all of its natural movements, including flexion (bending

BELLY BULGE

✳

The surest sign of abdominal weakness is the dreaded belly bulge. Not only will you develop a permanent pot belly, but working with a belly bulge leaves your low back vulnerable to strain and eventually pain if you continue to train that way.

the body forward), extension (arching the body back), and rotation (twisting the body). A strong center stabilizes the muscles of your hips and helps keep your pelvis in place. It reduces the workload on your limbs and lessens the strain on injury prone areas, such as your lower back and delicate shoulder joints, helping to prevent injury. With a strong center you will improve your posture so you stand a little taller. And of course, you'll have fabulous abs!

Once you learn how to tap into your center for extra power, this strength can come in handy in your everyday life. Strong upper back muscles stabilize your shoulders and help keep them in place, so you can activate your upper back to help reduce the work load for your arms. You can actually learn to move your arms from your upper back. Strong lower back muscles and abdominals help in the same way. They stabilize your pelvis and help keep it in its place so you can move from your powerhouse to lessen the workload for your legs in all kinds of activities, from walking and running to bending and lifting. Easy and efficient movement flows out from your center.

GUIDING PRINCIPLE FOUR: FLOW

When you center your body and concentrate on the exercise, all motion will flow smoothly and evenly from your center—not too fast or too slow. As you move through your motions, watch for jerky movements or motions where you gut stuck and can't perform the exercise correctly. If you do, modify! Furthermore, don't rush through the exercises to "get-your-workout-over," rather focus on lengthening your arms and legs from a strong center—I say, "Imagine *long and luscious,* and you will be *long and luscious.*"

GUIDING PRINCIPLE FIVE: PRECISION

As these principles come together, so should your mind and movement, creating a balanced body from within. Precision makes difficult exercises seem easy. Imagine an elite athlete, such as Lance Armstrong. He makes riding a bike over the steep mountains of France look easy in the *Tour De France* when, in fact, we all know how treacherous the terrain is. Precision creates grace in the movement, as you effortlessly flow from step to step. Joseph Pilates said, "Correctly executed and mastered to the point of sub-conscious reaction, these exercises will reflect grace and balance in your routine activities."

GUIDING PRINCIPLE SIX: BREATHING

"Even if you follow no other instructions, learn to breathe correctly," said Joseph Pilates. With every conscious breath, you will feel healthier and look better, and combined with concentration, mindful breathing will help you find your focus. Your breath helps strengthen your center, preserving the integrity of each exercise, and breaks the cycle of stress, calming you in the process. There is impressive research stating that breathing techniques can help overcome various health conditions that feed on stress, including heart disease and high blood pressure.

Life's Precious Nutrient: Your Breath

Your respiratory system, including your nose, mouth, windpipe, and all parts of your lungs and diaphragm, deliver life's most precious nutrient—oxygen. Your lungs work like two balloons that sit secure in your rib cage, expanding and deflating. Between each rib are muscles called the internal and external intercostals. As you inhale and exhale, these intercostals open and close your rib cage, working in conjunction with your diaphragm as it pumps air in and out of your lungs. When you inhale, your diaphragm relaxes and pushes downward to create a vacuum-like suction, drawing air into your lungs. To expel the air, it rises up pushing air out of your lungs. Breathing gives you so much more, including:

* Exchanging oxygen and carbon dioxide within the cells of your body.

* Carrying nutrients to every part of your body. Breath is the fuel for your body's cells, which need oxygen to thrive and produce the energy necessary to carry out various biochemical duties.

* Cleansing the toxins from your body. Toxin overload can leave you feeling tired and blah. Your lungs help get rid of emotional and physical toxins.

* Calming you down when life's twists and turns throw you a curve ball.

* Helping you to sharpen your concentration.

* Pumping you up to get you ready for the performance of your life.

* Strengthening your powerhouse.

It's not enough to just breathe, you must pay attention to your breath. Joseph Pilates said, "Squeeze every atom of impure air from your lungs in much the same manner that you would wring every drop of water from a wet cloth."

The Pilates Breath

In Pilates, you will practice back, or lateral, breathing. The idea is to breathe deeply enough to exchange dead air for fresh air so you feel vibrantly alive, and to increase your breathing capacity. In order to fill your lungs, imagine growing from within to open each rib in your back. Then exhale by pulling your navel to your spine, emptying every ounce of air from your lungs. Your abdominals will help facilitate a deep inner pull as they get stronger, helping you to feel a tightening sensation around your waist on deep exhalations.

Even though you will have plenty of practice in the next chapter, try a few breaths now. Wrap your fingers around your rib cage, thumbs on your back ribs and fingers on your front ribs. Inhale through your nose, counting to three—feel the air enter through your nose, traveling down your throat and spine while opening each rib in your back, flaring your rib cage to the side and spreading your fingers. Do not worry if you cannot expand your ribs to the sides at first, you might have some muscle restriction due to pent up tension, which can block and decrease your breathing capacity. Your breath will improve with Pilates practice. As you exhale, open your mouth slightly and relax your tongue and jaw, emptying your lungs as if you are blowing out 100 candles on your birthday cake. While exhaling, pull your navel to your spine. Remember, as the strength of your abdominals increase, you will feel an inward-pulling sensation.

To accentuate the exhale, Joseph Pilates invented a breathometer, which was a pinwheel connected to a straw. He held this breathometer out in front of his clients and only would be satisfied with their exhale if they could make the pinwheel spin. As crazy as it may sound, the breathometer became a vital tool in the development of lung capacity.

This deep exhalation protects your spine as the deep, stabilizing muscles of your trunk tighten around your spine. In fact, the surest sign that you are not breathing correctly (and of abdominal weakness) is if your belly bulges. To eliminate this kind of belly bulge, inhale deeply to open your ribs and exhale completely to flatten your belly as much as possible; otherwise, you may develop a permanent pot belly. Working with a belly bulge leaves your lower back vulnerable to strain and eventually pain if you continue to train that way. This breath work takes time and patience, so begin practicing now. Follow these rules:

* Keep your breath flowing—never hold your breath.

* Inhale through your nose to expand your back and lateral ribs. Your inhalation is the inspiration for the movement.

* Exhale through your mouth as if you are blowing out 100 birthday candles. Remember, make Joseph Pilates proud— spin that pinwheel.

* When rotating or twisting, first inhale to grow tall in the spine, then exhale into the actual twist.

Words of Wisdom: Perfecting Pilates

To make your Pilates performance better in every way, you need to have some knowledge of a few common phrases. As you travel beyond this book, you will hear these words again and again. Keep in mind, though, that these words are meant only for guidance— they do not mean that your body is ready to follow them to the letter. You may, for example, not be able to touch your toes. Or maybe your abdominals are not strong enough to hold your head up properly, causing neck strain. Perhaps you cannot inhale deeply yet. Whatever the case, it's best not to force your body into a position it does not want to be in. This is where good judgment comes in. If you cannot physically execute an exercise or hold your body in a correct position—right down to the smallest detail— then you need to figure out why. Work toward mending whatever that issue is, whether that means modifying an exercise or completely eliminating it for the time being.

You will see the following phrases repeated throughout this book. Learn them now and you will feel prepared and confident about attending a traditional group mat class in the future.

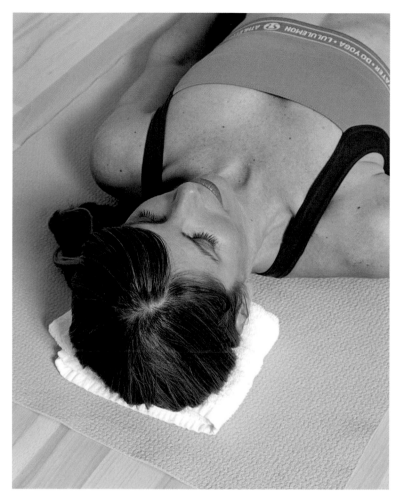

✳ CHIN TO CHEST is a phrase indicating proper head placement.
Mastering this position is especially important because the
majority of Pilates exercises require it. It does not involve
forcing your chin to your chest, rather a lengthening in the
back of your neck, which is actually an extension of your spine.
Imagine a swan's neck—long and lithe.

Try this: Place a towel under your head and let your shoulders
fall to the floor. Now gently guide your chin toward your chest.
This position will lengthen your spine, send awareness to your
upper spine, and is a safe position for your head and neck to
work in.

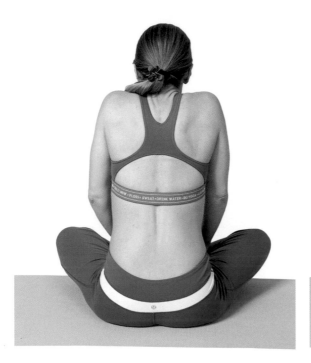 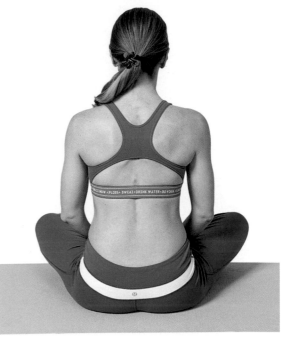

✳ DROPPING YOUR SHOULDERS helps relieve chronic tension that comes from holding your shoulders up and tight. By sliding your shoulder blades down your upper back and securing them in their proper place, you are also facilitating shoulder girdle stability and strengthening the muscles of your upper back and shoulders. When these muscles are strong, you might eventually free your chest and do away with a permanent state of hunched shoulders.

✳ LENGTHENING is a word used to describe stretching your limbs away from your center as if you are the tallest person in the world—*long and luscious!*

* PILATES BOX means working in the frame of your body. To work safely in your body and perform joint-friendly movements, your arms and legs should not extend past your shoulder and hip joints. With proper joint alignment, your limbs can move safely in a wide variety of movements without stressing your joints.

* PILATES STANCE describes how you will work with your legs. It is a foot position that places the heels of your feet together while your toes open about two to three fingers apart, forming a "V." This turn out begins at the hip bones and lengthens down your inner thighs so they are connected and your knees and ankles touch—imagine a magnetic force pulling your inner thighs together. The Pilates V will tone your inner thighs and buttocks, strengthen your pelvic floor muscles, and stabilize your lower body.

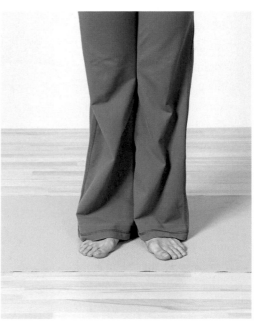

* RIBS TO HIPS is a phrase meaning drop your rib cage to your hips. Sometimes muscle tightness or weakness allows your rib cage to lift toward the ceiling, which also can cause an arch in the low back, throwing off your spine. You will drop your ribs to your hips to help center your body before any movement and, most importantly, to strengthen your abdominals correctly.

✳ SCOOPING is a word used to center your work by engaging your abs so your belly does not bulge. Scooping is used in conjunction with "navel to spine" or "scoop your belly button in and up." I like to use the phrase "hug your abs to your spine." Scooping takes place during a deep exhalation. Obviously, scooping your belly button up and in under your rib cage so your middle flattens takes a fair amount of abdominal strength. Be patient! Imagine slithering into your skinny jeans and zipping them up. Scooping your belly facilitates strengthening your deep abdominals, improves your movement, and goes hand-in-hand with rolling and unrolling your spine—bone by bone, stretching your lower spine.

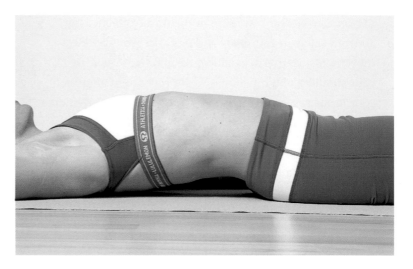

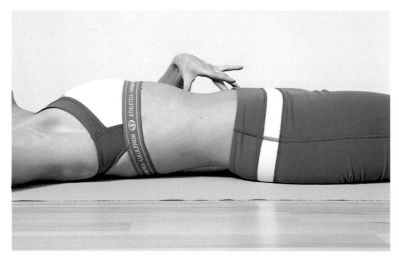

If you do not bring your belly button up and in, your lower back can leave the floor, which compromises your neutral spine and can result in low back strain and injury.

Notice the "scoop" as the navel draws to the spine, maintaining a neutral spine. You can place your fingers on your stomach to feel the change as you scoop your navel up and in.

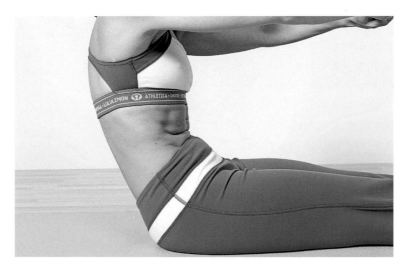

✳ SPINAL ARTICULATION means moving your spine vertebra by vertebra, or simply bone by bone. Whenever you read the phrase "spinal articulation," it means that you are moving one vertebra at a time to roll up to a sitting position or roll down to the floor. Moving bone by bone will stretch your spine, improve your spinal flexibility, nourish your spinal discs, and give you a better awareness of your pelvis.

✳ STRETCHING YOUR NECK describes proper head placement while your head is on the floor. It's creating length in the back of the head, neck, and shoulders, so your chin nears to your chest, as opposed to lifting your chin to the ceiling, which creates a severe arch in your cervical spine (your neck).

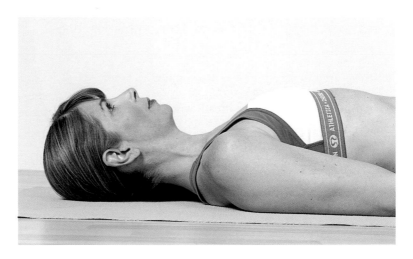

Fusing Mind and Motion: Principles in Use

Let's put these principles in practice by doing a simple exercise—a leg lift. Ordinarily, you probably lift your leg without much thought. But now, you will put these principles and phrases to good use by fusing your mind and body. Only then will these exercises become thoughtful motions. Remember, concentrate on even the smallest detail, so no motion is ignored. Check in with your body by centering it, and do not forget to breathe.

* Lie on your back with your legs extended. Place your hands at your sides.

* Lift your leg to the ceiling.

* Lower it to the floor.

What happened? Did you engage your mind? Were you able to lift your leg in the first place? Did you notice anything different, such as a pain, twinge, or pop? Here are some problems I've observed in my classes:

* When the leg lifts or lowers, the belly bulges as the lower back lifts from the floor.

* When the leg lowers, shoulders rise and bodies get scrunched up.

* The chin lifts toward the ceiling which can strain the delicate cervical spine—some students bunch up around the head, neck, and shoulders while lifting—others while lowering—their leg.

* Knees are often bent or legs are crooked.

* Many students hold their breath when lifting their leg or lowering it.

Some of the above limitations are due to a lack of strength, flexibility, and body knowledge. Of course, as you begin to study your body (you will do a variety of awareness exercises in chapter 3) and become familiar with its strengths and weaknesses, then you can begin to correct yourself and work with proper alignment. Here is your first lesson in body movement—doing it the Pilates way.

* Lie flat on your back with your legs extended and your arms at your sides.

* Check in with your body and ask yourself how you feel and if your body is aligned—a one minute body review will help you concentrate on what you are about to do.

* Center your body by dropping your navel to the floor so your center feels anchored to the floor. Do not lose your centering throughout the motion.

* Drop your shoulders away from your ears by lengthening your fingertips toward your toes, pressing the back of your shoulders into the floor.

* Lower your chin toward your chest so the back of your neck is long.

* Inhale so every rib opens.

* Exhale to lift your leg to the ceiling.

* Inhale and reach your toes out from your center, lengthening both your legs.

* Exhale to lower your leg to the floor, centering at all times.

Did you feel a difference doing the exercise this way? What changed? The Pilates way puts a new spin on an old exercise and gets you to work safely in your own body.

CENTERING:

A guiding principle requiring that you center your body before beginning any exercise.

CHIN TO CHEST:

A phrase describing proper head positioning.

CONCENTRATE:

A guiding principle encouraging you to find your focus.

CONTROL:

A guiding principle requiring you to move in control.

DROP YOUR SHOULDERS:

A phrase describing proper shoulder placement. Bring your shoulders down to relieve tension, lengthen your neck, and engage the correct muscles in your upper body.

FLOW:

A guiding principle requiring that all motion flows from your center.

LENGTHENING:

A term used to describe stretching your limbs as long as possible.

PILATES BREATH:

A phrase describing proper breathing. Inhale into your back ribs, expanding your rib cage laterally, and forcibly exhale to drop your navel to your spine.

PILATES BOX:

A phrase reminding you that your arms and legs should work within the boundaries of your shoulder and hip joints.

PILATES STANCE OR V:

A phrase describing proper foot placement with your feet turned out slightly. This optimal leg position lets you engage your inner thighs, buttocks, and pelvic floor muscles.

POWERHOUSE:

A term that Joseph Pilates coined meaning your center. Joseph Pilates also called your center your "girdle of strength."

PRECISION:

A guiding principle defining ease of movement and economy of movement.

RIBS TO HIPS:

A phrase describing proper rib placement: Your stomach muscles should engage to bring your ribs toward your hips, rather than lifting to the ceiling causing your lower back to arch.

SCOOP:

A term used in conjunction with "navel to spine"; your belly should never bulge.

SOFT FOOT:

A phrase describing a natural, relaxed foot position.

STRETCH YOUR NECK:

A phrase describing proper head and neck placement when your head is down on the mat. Do not lift your chin to the ceiling, which creates a severe arch in your cervical spine.

Fusing your mind and motion will guide you toward moving with ease, confidence, and poise in your private life as well as your fitness. My hope is that you will integrate your life on and off the mat.

* * *

One of the essential goals of Joseph Pilates' work (besides tightening and toning) is to create a fusion of your mind and body so that eventually your movements will come naturally without thinking about proper alignment.

* * *

The six guiding principles that fuse your body and mind are interrelated to move you safely in motion: concentration, control, centering, flow, precision, and breathing.

* * *

Good breathing will help your performance, reduce your stress, increase your stamina, and detoxify your body.

* * *

Joseph Pilates called your torso the "girdle of strength," which is why every exercise begins with centering.

* * *

All Pilates exercises coordinate your breath with the motions to improve breath awareness and enhance your execution.

* * *

Joseph Pilates believed that full deep breaths rid your body of toxins that make you feel blah and zap the zest from your life.

* * *

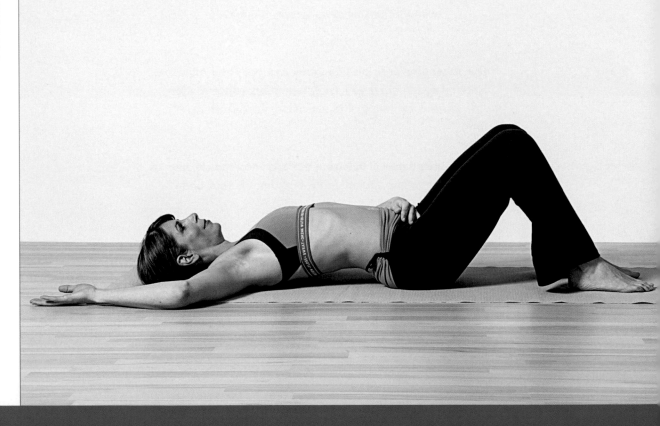

CHAPTER THREE

SOOTHE AND MOVE

AFTER CLASS ONE DAY, one of my students said, "Karon, I heard your voice replaying in my head while I was lifting weights—Shoulders down! Spine tall! Belly in!" As she repeated my words, I thought, "Wow, they really do listen to me." And while I beamed with pride, I feel this is really a testament to how versatile Pilates is.

My students want a good workout, buy I also try to strike a balance between the movements themselves and the reason for doing them. Pilates in not just a vast body of exercises, it is a philosophy for a healthy life. Yes, I can recite the exercises by heart, but if this is all I did in class, my students would never know what Pilates fully embodies.

This chapter will introduce you to the guts (literally) of Pilates so you can evolve toward healthier movement. You will first learn some basic fundamentals and then incorporate them in a series of awareness exercises to retrain your muscles. You'll develop a deeper understanding of your own body's complexities, which will allow you to advance as you continue your practice.

THE PLAN

The first step is to create a new mental environment. These movements are not big or fast, but subtle and very deliberate so as to allow deep muscle retraining to take place. It is not enough to know that you hold tension in your shoulders—you must make a conscious effort to relax them. Awareness will change your patterns of movements on or off the mat.

To ease you into these exercises and guide you toward healthier movements, you will need a yoga belt, a small hand towel, a medium-sized pillow, and a mat.

YOUR GOALS FOR CHAPTER THREE:

awareness exercises

* Reprogram your movements so you will train safely and prevent overstraining in delicate injury-prone areas, such as your low back.

* Learn how to engage your mind while exercising by doing a body scan of key areas of your body.

* Coordinate your breath with your movements. Concentrate on your motions without holding your breath. Discover areas of tightness in your body and then use your breath, specifically an *extended exhalation*, to relax tight muscles and ease stress.

* Recognize muscular imbalances. For example, if one shoulder is higher than the other, then you may have a muscular imbalance.

* Develop body symmetry between muscles.

* Ease overused muscles, which are more prone to injury. For example, most people with low back pain believe that their backs are weak, when in fact their backs are overworked.

* Build strength and awareness to progress to chapter 4.

SEQUENCE OF EXERCISES
SOOTHE AND MOVE

*

BREATHING LESSONS

FINDING A NEUTRAL PELVIS

PELVIC CLOCKS

KNEE FOLDS

KNEE STIRS

LEG SLIDES

OPEN LEGS TO SIDES

SHOULDER DROPS

RIB STRETCH

RIB CAGE ARMS

NOSE CIRCLES

TOWEL ROLL UP

HEAD ROLL UP

Breathing Lessons

Remember, your breath is the inspiration for each exercise; it pre-
pares you for the motion and will help you work in harmony with
your body to facilitate physical and emotional change. Because
breath plays a principle and intricate part in changing your body,
you will begin with breathing lessons. To begin, cinch your yoga
belt around the bottom half of your rib cage. This will help you
feel the opening and closing of your ribs while your lungs take in
and let out air. Use this awareness to establish a deep flow of air to
all parts of your lungs and to fine tune your Pilates breath.

B R E A T H I N G   L E S S O N   O N E
DIAPHRAGMATIC BREATHING

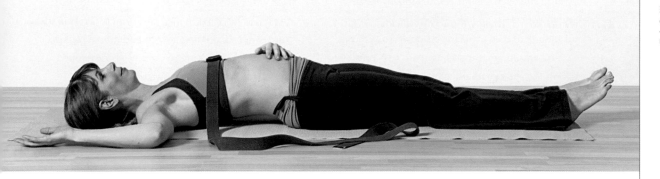

1. Lie on your back with your legs straight out or in
   any comfortable position. Put your hands on your
   belly and breathe normally. For the next few minutes, just relax and observe your natural breath.
   Your belly will rise and fall. You may notice some
   restriction or perhaps your breath is uneven and
   erratic when you try to deepen your breath. Or
   perhaps your breath is quick and choppy. This is
   the time to observe your breath and nothing
   more. Have you ever watched a baby sleep—her
   tummy rising and falling effortlessly? That is your
   goal, to belly breathe and deepen your breath.

2. If you feel that your breath is blocked, try to
   lengthen your exhalations, which might help
   relieve pent up emotional tension. Keep in mind
   that the depth of your breath is unconsciously
   controlled by your emotions; therefore, unre-
   solved emotions affect breathing. For example,
   chest breathing is a common protective response
   to pain, anguish, and anger. So, try to refocus
   your breath, extending the exhale a little more to
   relax you and let your emotional body feel secure
   enough to release whatever may be causing you
   to hold on to your tightness.

THE PILATES BREATH

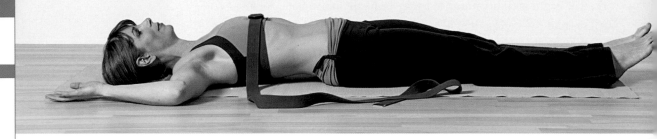

1 After several minutes of observing your belly rise and fall with your breath, begin to direct your breath to the back of your ribs. Gradually inhale through your nose and observe as the air relaxes your tongue and jaw and travels down your throat and into your lungs, expanding them as it opens each rib. As you breathe deeply, the belt will cinch around your rib cage. Imagine an inner tube as it fills with air, only it's your lungs opening rib by rib until they flare out to the side. At that point, your belly should not rise but flatten as you guide the air into the back ribs. Your belly should never bulge. If it does, then that is a sign of weakness or imbalance in your abdominal muscles.

2 Without hurrying, empty your lungs of air. Imagine that the inner tube has a slow leak. As each rib closes, the belt will loosen around your rib cage. This lengthened exhalation protects your spine while facilitating a deep abdominal muscle contraction. With practice and newly-developed strength, your abdominal wall will fall to the floor—navel to spine.

WORDS FROM JOSEPH PILATES

—————————— ✳ ——————————

"To breathe correctly you must completely exhale and inhale, always trying very hard to "squeeze" every atom of impure air from your lungs in much the same manner that you would wring every drop of water from a wet cloth."

Internal Girdle

Much of what you will do in Pilates focuses on creating a stable spine and pelvis by strengthening your trunk muscles. These muscles are arranged in layers that not only stabilize your spine but allow it to move. A few muscles, however, really stand out to form an internal girdle. Your deepest abdominal muscle, the transversus abdominis or transverse, provides a girdle of support for your spine by wrapping low around your waist as a seatbelt would.

The multifidus is a long and deep back muscle running from the sacrum to the cervical vertebrae. The multifidus' primary duty is to stabilize your spine and assist with extension (arching) and rotation (twisting).

The pelvic floor muscles assist in pelvic and spinal stability. Collectively, your pelvic floors make a sling or hammock of muscles that run in two different directions, from your pubic bone to tailbone and from one butt-bone to the other, to support the weight of your organs.

Now you know what I meant by "guts"! In every exercise, you will strive to engage your deep stabilizing muscles, or guts—imagine pulling up through your pelvic floors deep within your center and pulling in your belly button, engaging these deep contractions with your exhalations. You can feel your belly pull in when your transverse engages around your waist, but the contraction of the multifidus is more subtle. You can feel the pelvic floors engage by stopping the flow of your urine; it's a lift between your legs similar to Kegel exercises. Ideally, lifting the pit of your abdomen should be a soft action (nothing forced or strained). Move your muscles, but not your bones—especially not your hip bones.

Several other important muscles form the multiple layers making up your trunk and allow movement in your spine. These include the oblique system, which is divided into two muscles: your internal oblique and your external oblique. These muscles allow you to twist and bend at the waist. The rectus abdominis is a long, shallow abdominal muscle extending from your pubic bone to your sternum. You can feel it engage as you bend forward at the waist. The back muscles are primarily responsible for extension of the spine. One of the most well-known is the erector spinae; it runs from the sacrum to the last two thoracic vertebrae, helping to extend your spine.

All these muscles together form your trunk and move the spine in all of its natural movements: flexion, extension, and rotation. They are key to your health and vitality. As Joseph Pilates once said, "You're as old as your spine is flexible."

Body Scan: Neutral Spine

Earlier, I suggested giving yourself a 60-second body review before moving your body. I call it a body scan. Why is this important? A body scan will help you to create awareness, break old habits (such as tilting your head to the right or elevating your shoulders), and align your body so you can work safely without injuring yourself. Before you can move your body, you must have a starting point. This point is called neutral spine, meaning your bones, ligaments, muscles, and discs are where they should be. This position puts the least amount of stress on your body. Neutral spine is also the definition of good posture. Since so much of Pilates is based on postural awareness, neutral is a good place to start in your body.

Your back has three natural curves: The first is the slight curve in your neck, called the cervical curve, which is made up of the first seven vertebrae; the second is the middle back or thoracic curve, which encompasses the next twelve vertebrae; and finally, the third curve, the lumbar or lower back curve, which is between the pelvis and spine. Despite the fact that it is only five vertebrae, your lower back holds most of your body weight. In addition, your back has two fused bones acting as one unit: Five sacral vertebrae make up the flat bone of the buttocks, or sacrum, and the coccygeal vertebrae are the non-movable bones of your tailbone. All of these curves should be aligned (and I will go over proper alignment in greater detail later) while you sit, stand, exercise, or carry out your day-to-day activities to help lessen the strain on your body—hence the term neutral spine.

Although your spine is a complex system of bones, ligaments, muscles, and nerves, you can learn how to move it without damaging your body. Your internal girdle assists in maintaining a neutral and stable spine and, therefore, directly influences the position of your spine and its attached bones and other body parts, such as muscles. It is the continuous natural curve of your spine that keeps your body flowing as a unit. For this reason, it is helpful to begin by body scanning or checking the placement a few vital areas in your body: hips, shoulders, neck, and head.

Hip and pelvis placement is vital to establishing a neutral spine. Your hips, in fact, form the foundation of the pelvis and your pelvis influences what your lumbar spine is doing and, therefore, your whole spine. Because your body is a closed chain system, meaning what happens in one part of the body will eventually effect and alter another part, it is vital that you begin by evaluating the position of your pelvis.

Your pelvis is a bowl-like structure composed of many bones and muscles, including your pelvic floors. Your pelvis absorbs the weight of your body and transfers that weight to your legs. In addition, your pelvis must also absorb the stress from your legs because your pelvis attaches your legs to your spine. In other words, your pelvis absorbs the bulk of your weight whether you walk or jump. To do this, your pelvis must stabilize itself in the position that puts the least amount of stress on your body to ease the workload of your lower back. This position is called a neutral (or stable) pelvis, which is one component of neutral spine.

FINDING A NEUTRAL PELVIS

1 Lie on your back with your knees bent. Place the palm of your hand on your hip bone and your fingers on your pubic bone. In a neutral position, your hand should rest flat.

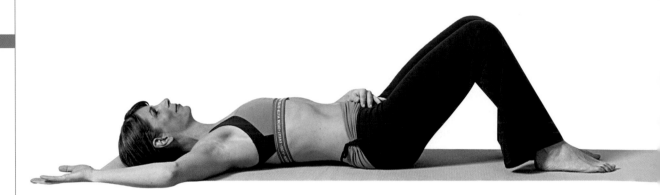

2 Inhale, then, on your exhale, gently pull your navel to your spine. Notice that your pubic bone tilts toward the ceiling and your lumbar spine flattens, letting no light shine through between your lower back and the floor. When your lower back is flat against the floor, your fingertips rise.

3 Inhale and move your pelvis so your tailbone drops to the floor. This position creates an extreme lumbar arch so light can shine between your lower back and the floor. In an extreme arch, the palm of your hand lifts higher than your fingers. Experiment by moving back and forth between these two positions and then end in a neutral spine— so the palm of the hand rest flat between those two bony points. Remember your abdominals move the bones of your pelvis!

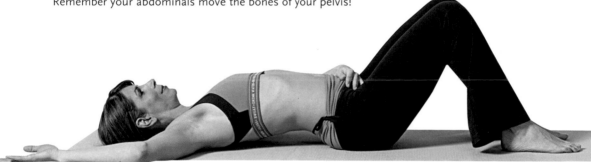

As you moved in and out of a neutral spine position, you were moving from one extreme curve (flattening) to another extreme curve (arching) of the lumbar spine. If your pelvis is locked in one of these extreme positions, then you could have some real back problems. In a neutral pelvis position, the pelvis and hip bones align in the middle of those two extreme positions to rest evenly— right where they should be!

PELVIC CLOCKS

With this mini-exercise, you will build awareness in your lower spine and hips and find weak areas in your abdominals and lower back muscles. It's also a nice stretch for your lower back. You should feel the pit of your belly dropping to your spine without moving your pelvic bones. Ideally, this inner pull is a subtle contraction—don't force it or press your low back into the mat.

Take a piece of paper and draw the face of a clock: 12:00, 3:00, 6:00, and 9:00. Take that piece of paper and place it over your pelvis, or just imagine your pelvis wearing a face of a clock: 12:00 rests on the end of the sternum, 6:00 is your pubic bone, 3:00 is your left hip bone, and 9:00 is your right hip bone .

6–12 CURL

1 Lie down on your back, with your knees bent. Place the palm of your hand on your low belly. Inhale, then, on your exhale, gently guide your navel to your spine and move into a 6:00–12:00 position. Notice your obliques drawing your ribs down and toward your hips while the pit of your belly sinks your navel to the floor.

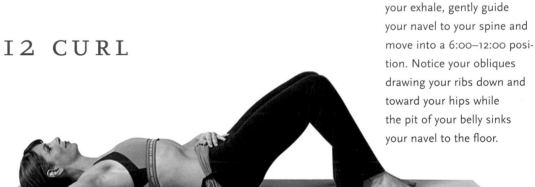

2 Inhale and move into a 12:00–6:00 position so your lower back arches—you should see a lot of light under your lower back. Repeat three to five times.

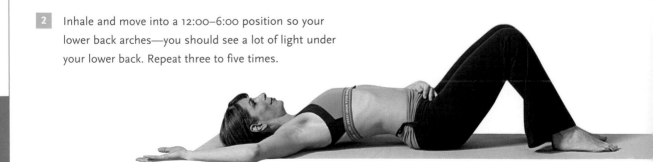

3–9 CURL

1   Inhale to lift your left hip and move your pelvis into the 3:00–9:00 position.

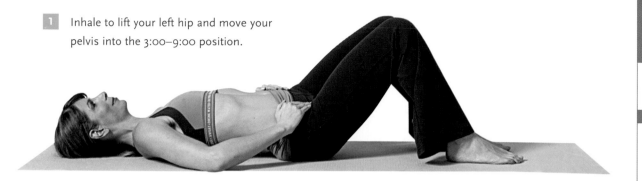

2   Exhale to neutral spine position while engaging your deep abdominals so the pit of your belly falls to the floor.

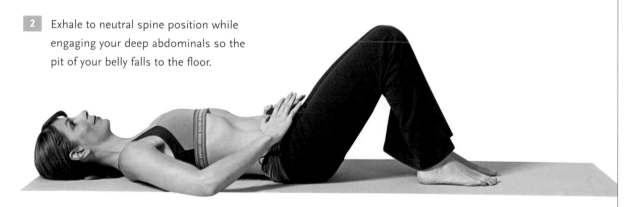

3   Inhale to lift your right hip and move your pelvis into the 9:00–3:00 position. As you move from side to side, try to maintain an even flow between both hip bones. Repeat three to five times.

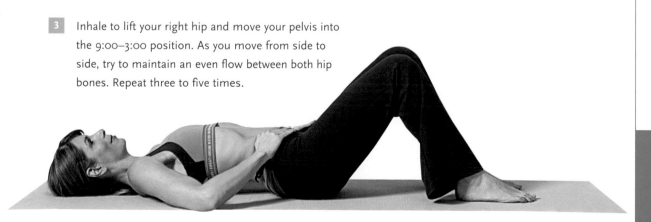

ROCK THE CLOCK

1 Inhale, then, on your exhale, scoop your abs toward the floor to initiate a hip circle.

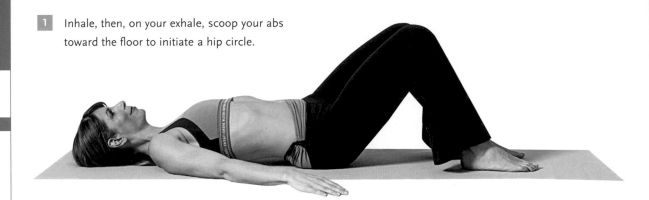

2 Lengthen your inhale as you lift your left hip bone into the 3:00–9:00 position and continue circling past the 12:00–6:00 position.

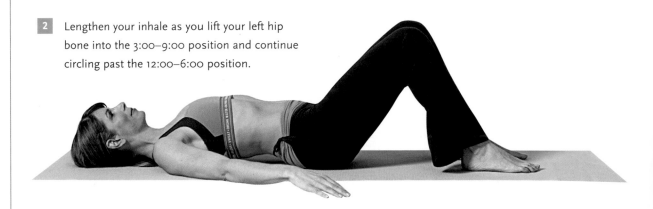

3 Exhale to lift your right hip bone and continue circling through the 9:00–3:00 position and continue past the 6:00–12:00 position, engaging your abs. Repeat three to five circles, then reverse directions.

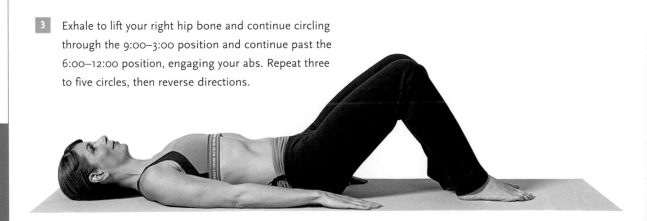

The next series of exercises help build awareness in your pelvis area and strengthen your abdominals. Most importantly, these exercises will teach you how to use your abdominals to move your legs while keeping your pelvis stable; it is important for your legs to move independently while your pelvis remains stable so you don't overwork and strain your low back. Protecting your lumbar spine is your priority.

✳

KNEE FOLDS

This exercise will teach you to maintain a neutral pelvis while moving your legs, challenge and strengthen your abdominals, and relieve lower back woes due to overstraining. Your goal is to fold your knee into your hip joint in a smooth motion (ease of movement) without disturbing your stable pelvis.

1 Lie on your back and bend your knees. Place your hands by your sides, palms down.

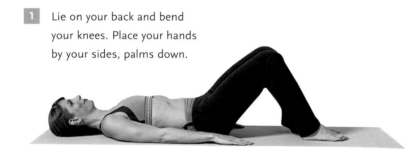

2 Inhale to mentally prepare for the movement, then, as you exhale, lift your right knee to a 90-degree angle so it's in line with your hips. Don't move your pelvis; it must remain in a stable (neutral) position. Return your leg to the floor without moving your pelvis. Repeat knee fold with your left leg.

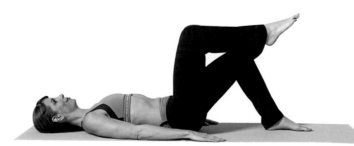

KNEE STIRS

This stretch will relieve tension in your hip joints and increase hip flexibility. Your goal is to become aware of your pelvis so you do not overuse your hip joints.

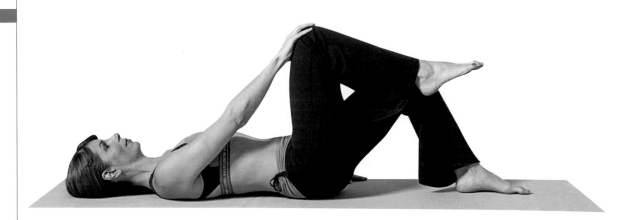

1 Lie on your back and bend your knees. With your right hand, pull your right knee to your chest. Notice if your hip leaves the floor in the process. The bones of your pelvis must remain even. If necessary, use your left hand to push your right hip bone down so it's even with the left—imagine that your hip is heavy and you can't lift it off the floor.

2 With your hand, gradually stir
your knee in its hip socket as
if it's a thick pot of chili.

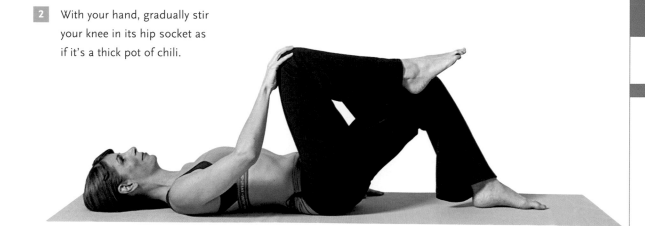

3 Continue circling your leg as
long as you want, then change
directions. Switch legs.

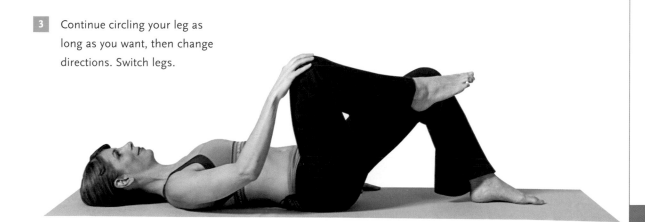

LEG SLIDES

This exercise will increase the challenge for your abdominals as you learn to keep your pelvis stable. As your leg stretches, so does a major hip flexor muscle called the psoas. Therefore, your abdominals must work harder to stabilize your pelvis. Keep in mind that as your leg slides out, your pelvis may arch, which disrupts your neutral position. To help keep your pelvis stable, focus on exhaling. Drop your navel to your spine to engage your transverse to assist in trunk stability. As the strength of your abdominals increase, you will have more control over your pelvis.

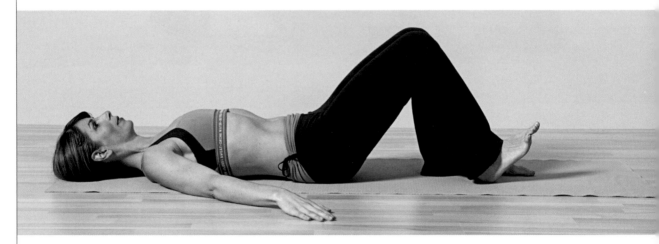

1 Lie down on your back with your knees bent. Place the palms of your hands on the bony points of your hips to help align them. After that, place your arms by your sides, palms down. Inhale to slide your heel away from your body.

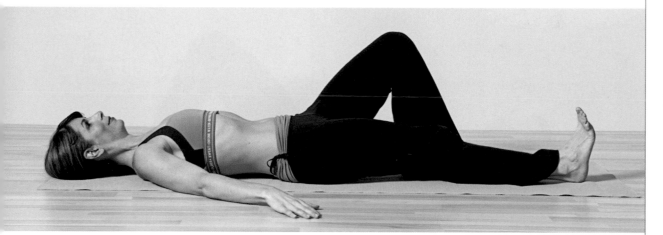

2 Continue to inhale as your leg straightens, then, as you exhale, slide your heel toward your bottom to bend your knee. Repeat three to five times for each leg.

OPEN LEGS TO SIDES

This exercise will coordinate your abdominals and adductors (inner thigh muscles) so that they can work together to stabilize your pelvis, engage your obliques, help improve hip flexibility, and relieve tension in your lower back. This time, your legs open to the side to challenge your pelvic stability. Try to establish a smooth flow as you open and close your legs. Keep in mind that any tightness in your inner thighs can affect the position of your pelvis because your adductors attach just below your pubic bone, which is why this exercise is an awareness exercise as well as a strengthening one.

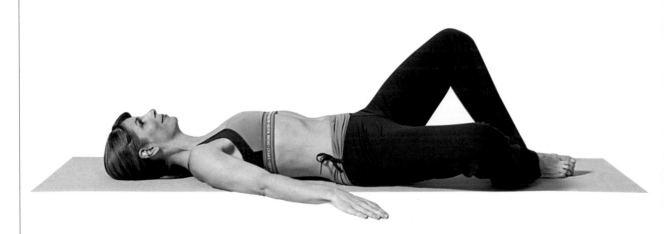

1 Lie on your back with your knees bent. Lengthen your arms by your sides. Inhale, then, on your exhale, open your right leg to the side. As your leg opens, your pelvis will want to shift with the weight of your leg. To offset this and help stabilize your pelvis, exhale and drop your navel to your spine. Focus on your ribs, keeping them down toward your hips to engage and strengthen your obliques. Repeat three to five times and then switch legs.

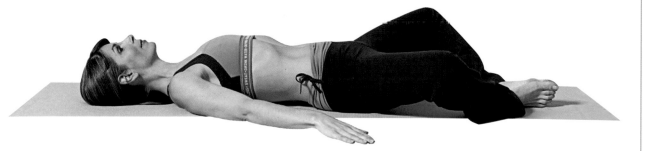

2 Return to the starting position, then open both legs at the same time. Remember, the obliques keep your ribs from lifting to the ceiling. Repeat three to five times.

Body Scan: Shoulders

As you work your way up your spine in your body scan, stop at your shoulders. Ask yourself: Is one shoulder higher than the other? Are my shoulders lifted as if I am tense or stressed? Do my shoulders round like my grandmothers? If so, you are not alone. Many people suffer from chronic tension and therefore suffer from chronic upper back tightness. You may also make matters worse by how you spend your day: Are you scrunched over a desk or computer? If so, this will further weaken the muscles supporting your upper spine.

Judging from my students, lack of awareness is part of the problem. In class, I say, "Drop your shoulders!" no less than fifty times during any given hour; it's a problem for the majority of my students. Dropping your shoulders seems easy enough, but chronic tightness can interfere with maintaining a relaxed shoulder position. What is important to know is that you have two winged bones, called your shoulder blades or scapulae, that float on your upper spine. Engaging them can help depress your shoulders! By sliding these bones down your back, your shoulders will drop as well. In fact, all movement of your arms should initiate from those bones.

Your shoulder area attaches your arms to your spine. Your shoulder blades—along with other joints and a variety of important, yet somewhat obscure, muscles—play a major role in this connection. Even the simplest task, such as writing, takes a joint effort between these groups so you can move your pencil. The shoulders blades move your shoulders in many directions and helps stabilize them; it's important to understand that your shoulder blades form the foundation for your arms, just like the pelvis forms the foundation of your spine. Stabilization of both these crucial areas helps you maintain a neutral spine.

To feel shoulder blade engagement, try this: Lift your shoulders to your ears and slightly back and then slide your shoulders blades down your back. You should feel a little taller, perhaps lifted, as your chest opens. Imagine that you have a set of deep pockets resting on your back, waiting for your shoulder blades to slide in for safekeeping.

If at first you find this difficult, then you may have a combination of muscle tightness or weakness in a variety of muscles. A combination of tight chest muscles and lengthened, weak upper back muscles can keep you in a permanent state of hunching. Another common problem is that the shoulder blades wing out so they do not rest flat against the spine. However, the most common problem by far is chronically high shoulders, perhaps due to your 9-5 job. A busy lifestyle with deadlines, a difficult boss, and lack of sleep, among other stresses, can all cause shoulder tension. This is where you can make some subtle changes in your own body. First, be aware of how you hold your shoulders. Then you can begin to retrain your body's movements, along with some of the muscles of your upper back.

Your shoulders enjoy lots of mobility and stability because a variety of specialized muscles allow your shoulder blades to move in a variety of directions. The primary muscles are the trapezius, or traps, which are a diamond-shaped muscle that originate on the base of your skull, attach to your shoulder blades, and end around the middle of your back. The rhomboids are relatively small; they sit on the spine of your upper back and between your shoulder blades. Then there is the serratus anterior, which is a thin muscle that originates on your lateral ribs and connects under your shoulder blades. Of course, there are many other muscles of the upper torso—think layers and layers of muscles. Some you probably know: The latissimus dorsi, or lats, extends from your lower spine to your upper arm bone. It is your biggest back muscle. The pectorals form the broad band of chest muscles. The deltoids are your shoulder muscles. These muscles all play an important role in keeping you moving and standing tall. Try a few of the following simple exercises.

SHOULDER DROPS

This exercise will release tension in your upper spine, warm up your shoulders, send awareness to your shoulder blades, and teach you how to move your shoulder blades on the thoracic spine. Remember, slide your shoulder blades into their pockets so movement can begin from there.

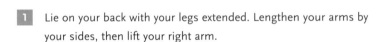

1 Lie on your back with your legs extended. Lengthen your arms by your sides, then lift your right arm.

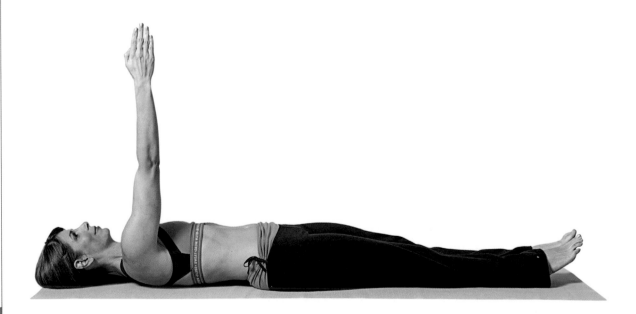

2 Inhale to stretch your fingertips to the ceiling, lifting the back of your shoulder off the floor. Exhale to drop the back of your shoulder to the floor while sliding your shoulder blade into its pocket. Melt every bone of your upper spine into the floor. Repeat three to five times and then switch arms.

RIB STRETCH

This exercise will move you into a deeper stretch for your upper spine, send awareness to the placement of your shoulder blades, and improve your shoulder flexibility.

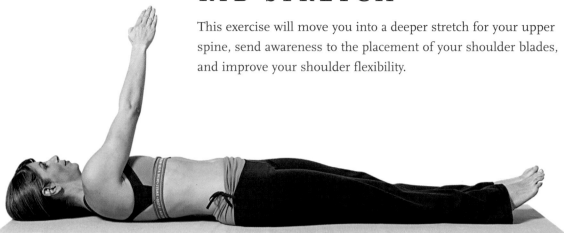

1 Lie on your back with your legs extended. Lengthen your arms by your sides. Inhale to lift your right arm to the ceiling and across your chest to initiate a stretch cross the upper spine. Take your arm higher and you will feel more rotation of your thoracic spine as well, which should feel great.

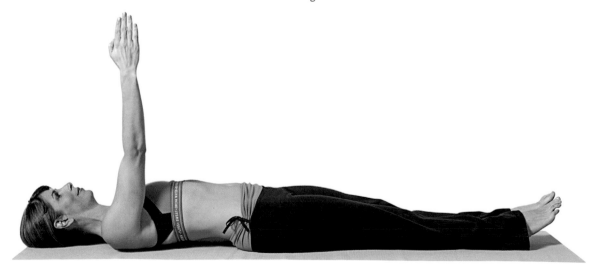

2 Exhale to lower your arm so the back of your shoulder falls to the floor—think heavy in your shoulders so they remain even and touch the floor. Try to make the movement come from your shoulder blade. Repeat three to five times and then switch arms.

RIB CAGE ARMS

This exercise will challenge your trunk stabilization, stretch your chest muscles, and strengthen your oblique abdominals. Keep in mind that as you lift your arms over your head, your rib cage will have a tendency to lift, especially if have tightness in your chest muscles, lats, or both. In any event, try to focus on your oblique abdominals to help keep your ribs down and your spine neutral. You should maintain "ribs to your hips" in just about every Pilates exercise, so it's important to pay attention to your rib placement.

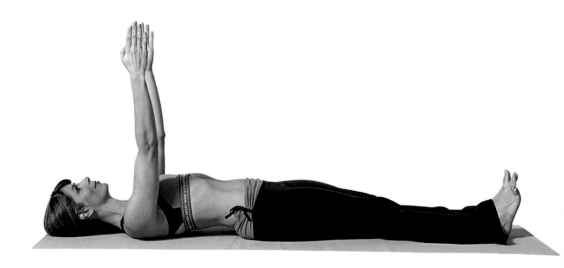

1 Lie on your back with your legs extended. Lift both of your arms to the ceiling, but keep your shoulders grounded to the floor.

2   Reach your arms over your head. Pay attention to your front ribs! Only take your arms to a point at which your ribs don't lift toward the ceiling and are close to your hips. This is important—if your ribs lift, then you're losing a vital source of your abdominal power from your obliques. Eventually, you'll have enough flexibility and strength to raise your arms completely over your head while keeping your "ribs to your hips."

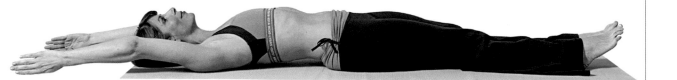

Body Scan: Lengthen your Neck

Your neck is made to be gently positioned in alignment with your spine. But because chronic neck tension is an epidemic in today's multi-tasking world, this connection is often severed, leaving you feeling tired, tense, and often headachy. It's important to approach your head and neck with great respect, because these muscles, soft tissues, and bones are delicate.

You should check your head and neck alignment before any movement to protect your cervical bones and establish neutral spine as well. Many of the Pilates exercises begin by curling your chin toward your chest and holding that position for some time; therefore, you must practice proper alignment so you do not strain these delicate muscles and bones. Keep in mind that lengthening through the back of the neck will help offset fatigue and poor alignment.

Your cervical spine should have a slight curve, but chronic tightness can alter this position and weaken a variety of muscle groups in the process. Neck issues can also originate from another part of your body—remember, what happens in one part of your body will eventually affect another part. Clenching your jaw, for example, can lead to poor head-neck alignment and more serious back problems. A key rule is to look at your whole spine from top to bottom in these early stages.

One more thing: If you cannot draw your chin to your chest, then do not force it! You must work cautiously with your neck, because you do not want to strain ligaments and muscles. As with any muscle, it will stretch naturally at its own pace. A few primary muscles of the neck are the levator scapulae, which extend from your neck vertebrae to each shoulder blade, and the upper trapezius muscles, which also attach to your shoulder blades and base of your skull and neck vertebrae—together these muscles bend your neck back. The sternocleidomastoid, which is the thick neck muscle in the front of your neck, flexes your neck; it assists in curling your chin toward your chest and moving your head from side to side. As I said earlier, most Pilates exercises begin by gently guiding your chin to your chest while lengthening the back of your neck. The following are awareness exercises that also build strength.

NOSE CIRCLES

This exercise will release tension in your neck and shoulders, open your cervical joints, and improve awareness of your neck-head alignment. Remember, chronic tightness can alter the alignment of the spine regardless of where it starts.

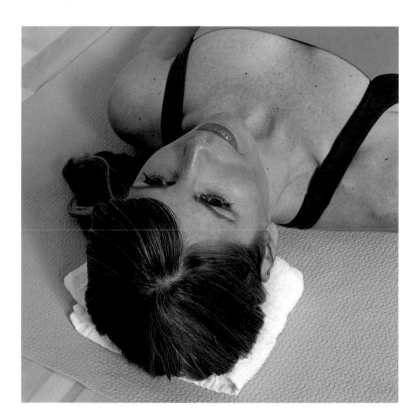

1 Lie on your back with your legs extended. Lengthen your arms by your sides. Close your eyes and relax. Ask yourself: Is my chin sticking up towards the ceiling, creating a severe arch in my neck? If so, there may be tightness somewhere. To help offset this tightness, place a small hand towel underneath the back of your head to give it a little lift. This way, you can work with proper neck-head alignment and it should feel much better on your neck as well. Focus on your Pilates breath while melting each bone of your spine into the floor. When you're ready, draw a tiny circle with the tip of your nose—imagine the size of the inner circle of a bagel. These circles should be small and smooth. Repeat three to five times and then reverse the circle.

TOWEL ROLL UP

This exercise will build strength in the muscles that curl your chin to your chest and lengthen the muscles in the back of your neck.

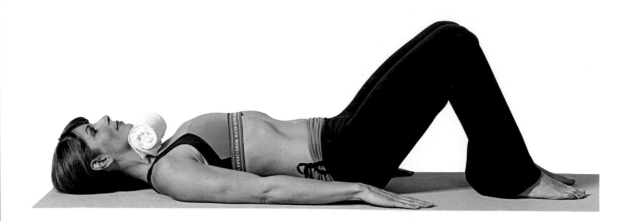

1 Lie on your back with your knees bent, feet hip-width apart and parallel. Lengthen your arms by your sides after placing a rolled up towel between your chin and throat. Gently lower your chin a bit and use your muscles to hold the towel in position. Stop here if you can't draw your chin to your chest—just relax with a pad under your head. You should naturally feel the muscles behind your neck stretching and lengthening while the deep neck flexors in the front are working to keep the towel in place—releasing the muscles of the back of your neck. If your neck veins are popping out, you're pushing too hard. Breathe and relax your jaw and tongue.

HEAD ROLL UP

This exercise will build strength in the muscles that curl your chin to your chest, lengthen the muscles in the back of your neck, and teach you how to begin each Pilates exercise.

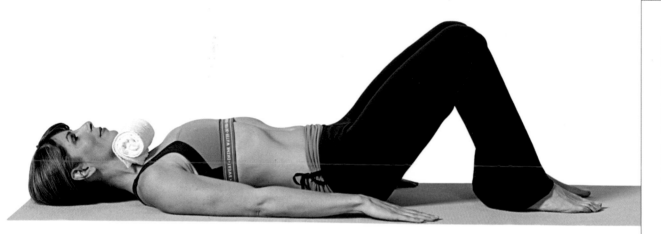

1 Lie on your back with your knees bent, feet hip-width apart and parallel. Lengthen your arms by your sides after placing a rolled up hand towel underneath your chin.

continued on next page ➤

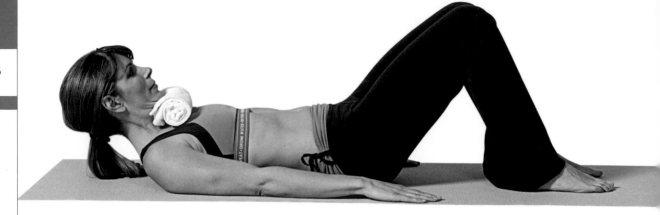

 With your arms extended by your sides, palms down, slide your fingers closer to your toes—sliding your shoulder blades into their pockets. Inhale to prepare for the movement, then, on your exhale, curl your chin to your chest to lift your shoulders slightly off the floor. As your chin moves closer to your chest, lengthen the back of your neck. Hold for two breaths, then lower your upper body. Repeat three to five times.

NECK PRECAUTION

❋

If you have any neck issues, please check with your doctor or physical therapist. If you get the okay, then begin by working with a pillow under your head for support. You can progress to working with a hand towel under your chin and then attempt the neck roll up. You should never feel any pain or strain in your neck when performing these exercises.

STRETCHING YOUR LIMITS

✳

These awareness exercises will retrain your muscles and how you eventually move them. You are not in any rush to advance. We all have many bad habits to unlearn and we all must learn how to take a gentler approach with our bodies. I hope these exercises leave you feeling as if you have learned a little about your own body—and feeling good about it. Below is your chapter review:

* * *

It's so important to look at your whole spine from top to bottom in these early stages. So do a body scan of your hips, shoulders, neck, and head.

* * *

Much of what you will do in Pilates focuses on maintaining a neutral spine and creating spinal and pelvic stability through the strength of your deepest muscles, the transversus abdominis, multifidus, and pelvic floors.

* * *

Chronic tightness can alter the connection between many muscle groups and joints. Neck issues can originate from another part of the spine—remember, what happensin one part of the spine will eventually affect another part.

* * *

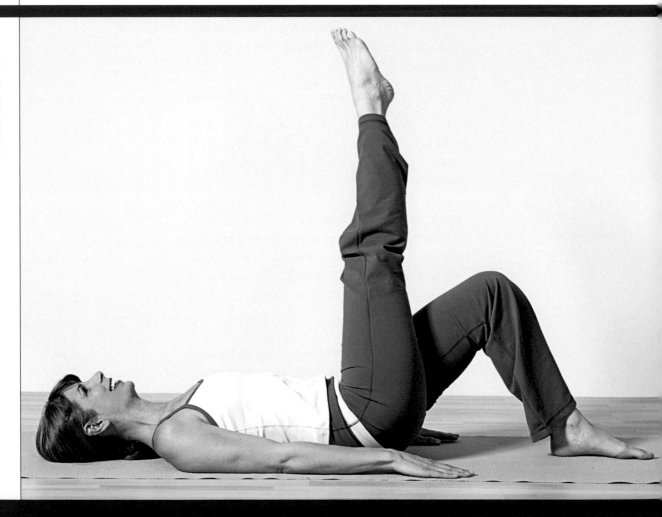

FIT AND LITE

HERE'S WHERE IT ALL BEGINS: total concentration, control of movement, centering your body, and connecting with your breath. In this chapter, you will explore your body to its fullest potential. And soon, you will discover how each of the Pilates fundamentals directly influences the exercises. Each exercise simulates classic Pilates exercises while focusing on the fundamentals so you will gain more strength, flexibility, and awareness in your own body. Stay in the moment and your body will thrive.

THE PLAN

Neuroscience has long proven that the brain programs the body—your mind teaches your muscles. These exercises, therefore, focus on what you have already learned and form the foundation for the classic Pilates mat exercises. Still, even in these early stages, begin to memorize these exercises and how to do them properly so you can progress with confidence, strength, and ease of movement. For this Fit and Lite workout, you will need a medium sized pillow, yoga belt, small hand towel, and a mat to protect your back. Stick with this workout for at least six weeks, doing it at least two to three days a week. Good luck and memorize these words—stable and scoop!

YOUR GOALS FOR CHAPTER FOUR:

level one

* Repeat this mental mantra: head, neck, shoulders, and hips! Do a 60-second body scan of these areas of your body to be sure you move with proper alignment at all times. You can do this mental scan as many times as you need to during each exercise.

* Focus on stabilizing your trunk and scooping your belly button up and in toward your spine—hugging your abs to your spine the whole time. Stable and scoop!

* Concentrate on your Pilates breath: During each inhalation open your ribs so they can expand laterally and then close each rib as you exhale—all of your effort is on the exhalation.

SEQUENCE OF EXERCISES
FIT AND LITE
✳

PILLOW SQUEEZE

THE FIFTY (ON WALL)

SNAKE LEGS

CURL DOWNS

HAMSTRING, ANKLE,
AND FOOT STRETCHES

LEG CIRCLES

BABY ROCKING

SINGLE LEG STRETCH
(WALL)

DOUBLE LEG STRETCH
(WALL)

PRONE BREATHING

PILLOW SQUEEZE
(PRONE)

LEG WORK

CHILD'S POSE

PILLOW SQUEEZE

This exercise will strengthen your inner thighs and pelvic floors, open your hip and sacroiliac joints, stretch your low back, and relieve low back tension, including any sacral pain. The strength of your pelvic floors is essential in trunk stabilization and for correct posture, so focus on pulling up through your center and inner thighs.

1 Lie on your back with your knees bent, feet hip-width apart. Place the pillow between your knees and then lengthen your arms by your sides, palms down. Inhale, then, as you exhale, squeeze the pillow between your knees. Maintain a stable pelvis while contracting your inner thighs.

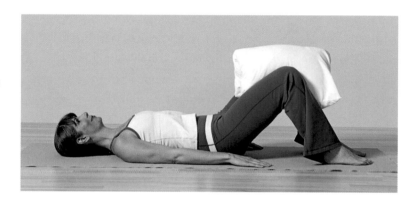

FUSING MIND AND MOTION

✳

Inhale to send your breath into your lateral ribs.

✳✳✳

Exhale to squeeze the pillow and feel the contraction between your thighs.

✳✳✳

Repeat five to eight times.

HEAD TO TOE ALIGNMENT TIPS

✳

1. Don't move your pelvis. The idea is to contract between your inner thighs, activating and strengthening your pelvic floor muscles.

2. Relax your upper body and focus on the contraction between your inner thighs and pelvic floor muscles.

THE FIFTY (ON WALL)

The Hundred is a classic Joseph Pilates exercise and is the first exercise you will do in a regular Pilates class. However, you will begin here with a reduced count of 50 until your abdominal strength improves. This exercise will warm up your body, stimulate your body's circulation, increase your breathing capacity, strengthen your abdominals, and is your first attempt at connecting your breath to the movement.

Your goals are several: stabilizing and lengthening your torso by melting each bone of your spine into the mat, learning to pump your arms correctly, curling your chin to your chest without creating any stress on your neck, and exhaling so deeply that you scoop your belly button up and in to activate your transverse.

Pay particular attention to the alignment of your spine and listen to how your body feels. In most new students, the neck flexor muscles (the ones on the front of your neck) have a tendency to tire first, causing neck strain. By placing your feet on the wall, you can help anchor your spine, which will also lessen the strain on your delicate neck muscles and the rest of your body as well.

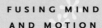

FUSING MIND AND MOTION

✳

You'll pump your arms deeply, about six to eight inches, to create resistance. Inhale for five counts and exhale for five counts, adding up to five full breaths and fifty arm pumps.

✳✳✳

If you can't inhale for five, then reduce your breath count to three and exhale for three. You will eventually be able to increase this count as your breathing capacity improves.

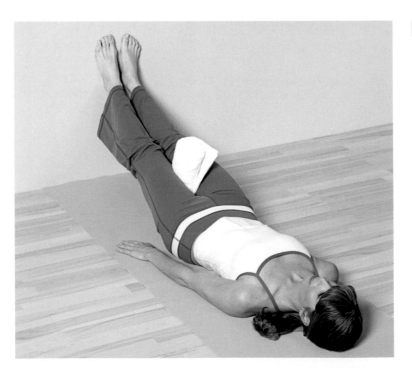

1 Lie on your back with feet hip-width apart. Place your hands by your sides, palms down. Walk your right foot up the wall and then your left foot, so that your legs are extended. Place a pillow or rolled up towel between your thighs. Relax and take a few breaths.

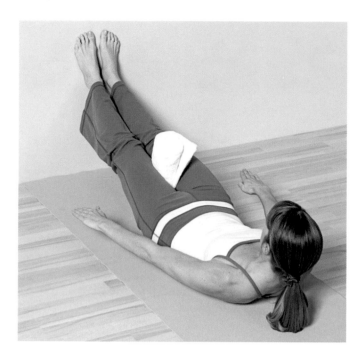

2 Curl your chin to your chest and begin to lift the palms of your hands off the floor about two inches, or until the back of your shoulders come off the floor. Stretch your fingertips to the wall. Inhale as you vigorously pump your arms up and down for a count of five, then, as you exhale, pump your arms up and down for another count of five. Imagine your arms pushing through sludge, creating resistance with each pump.

HEAD TO TOE ALIGNMENT TIPS

✳

1. If you have any neck issues, please talk to your doctor before doing the Hundred (or, in this case, the Fifty). Even without neck problems, your neck may tire before your body does. It's not uncommon for the muscles of your neck to be weak. This causes overstraining as you struggle to hold your head up, particularly if you have a misalignment of your cervical spine. Be careful with your delicate neck muscles. You can place a pillow behind your head for support at any time and then continue the exercise. Or, you can place one hand behind your head for support. You can always lower you head to the mat if needed.

2. Don't bounce your torso as you pump your arms up and down. Stabilize your body by placing your feet against the wall and focus on squeezing the towel between your legs.

3. While pumping, exhale every last ounce of air out of your body, scooping your navel up and in under your rib cage and toward your spine.

4. After the Fifty, keep your feet on the wall.

SNAKE LEGS

This stretch will help free the hip joints, relieve some low back tension, stretch your inner thighs and groin muscles, and send awareness to your pelvis. Enjoy this stretch—it's soothing.

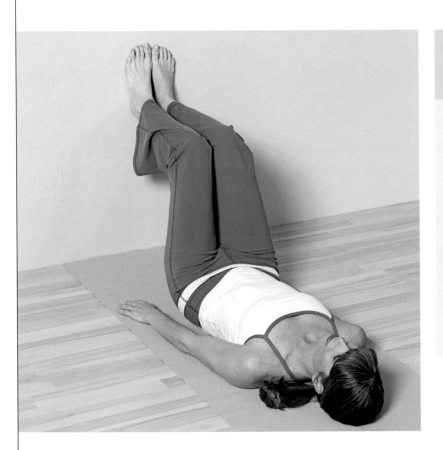

FUSING MIND AND MOTION

✳

This is a feel good stretch, but it can also provide helpful information about muscle imbalance. If you have tightness or lack strength in your thighs, one leg may walk down the wall more quickly than the other. Pay attention here—muscle imbalance can eventually be corrected with awareness.

✳✳✳

Repeat three to five times.

1   Lie on your back with your knees bent, feet hip-width apart. Lengthen your arms by your sides, palms down. Walk your right foot up the wall and then your left foot, so your knees are at a 90-degree angle to your hips (knees directly over hip bones).

Relax and take a few breaths.

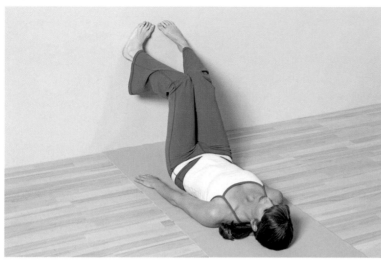

2 Walk your heels out so your toes and knees point in, facing one another.

3 Now move your toes out so your toes and knees point out to the side.

4 Follow this pattern until your legs are completely open, knees facing in. Reverse the walk.

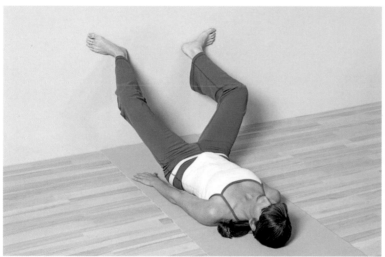

HEAD TO TOE ALIGNMENT TIPS

✳

1. You may feel that your movements are not flowing evenly between your legs. Send your awareness to that sticky spot, especially if you feel some tightness, and breathe to relax your muscles.

2. One leg may stray in a crooked manner while the other remains in line. Take this time to pay attention to your legs. Ask yourself: Is one leg tighter than the other, or perhaps stronger than the other?

3. Breathe normally.

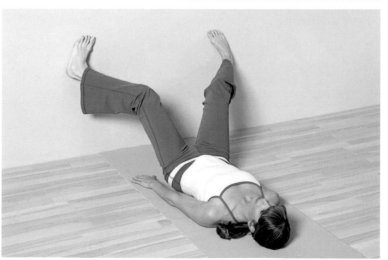

CURL DOWNS

This exercise will strengthen your abdominal muscles, begin to teach you how to roll down using spinal articulation, and stretch your spine by engaging your abdominals. As you learn how to curl your spine—imagine a string of pearls lowering to the floor—focus on exhaling fully to melt each bone to the mat.

FUSING MIND AND MOTION

*

Inhale to lower your chin to your chest, looking past your toes.

* * *

Exhale to curl your pubic bone to the ceiling and hollow your belly.

* * *

Continue to exhale as you curl down, lowering your spine to the mat bone by bone.

* * *

Repeat five to eight times.

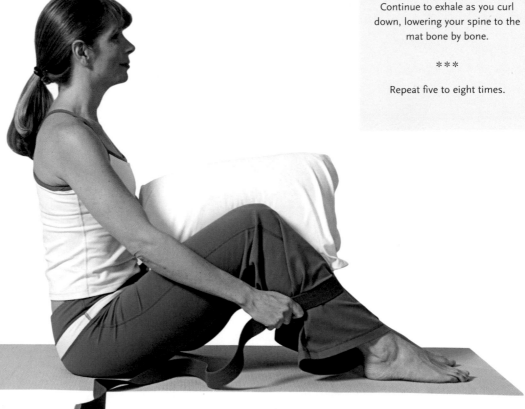

1 Sit on the floor with your knees bent, feet hip-width apart and firmly grounded to the floor. Place a pillow between your legs and wrap your yoga belt around your shins just below your knees. Hold the belt tight.

HEAD TO TOE ALIGNMENT TIPS

✳

1. If you have any back issues, consult you doctor. You may want to leave this exercise out if you have any back pain.

2. Relax your jaw and mouth and keep the back of your neck long.

3. Don't plop your body down. Focus on the deep scoop as you squeeze the pillow and don't forget to use the strap to help lower yourself to the floor safely.

4. Squeeze the pillow to engage your inner thighs and pelvic floors, which will help activate your stabilizing muscles.

5. Not only will you gain strength from this exercise, but you will learn how to maintain length in the front of your body. Remember, curl down—not crunch. So, curl and scoop, curl and scoop as a string of pearls lower to the mat.

6. Don't bulge your belly. Remember, the pit of your belly hollows to lengthen from the pubic bone to the navel. You will also feel a nice lower back stretch.

REMEMBER YOUR TRANSVERSE

✳

If your belly bulges at any point, then you're no longer working your transverse. The rectus abdominus (the most superficial muscle) has taken over, which might result in a permanent bulge if you continue to train with poor form— no loaf of bread in the belly!

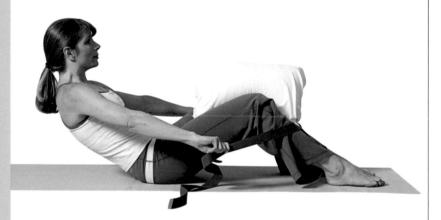

2 Inhale for inspiration, then, as you exhale, scoop your belly and squeeze the pillow to curl down, bone by bone, to the floor. Use the belt to guide you to the floor, letting it slide through your hands for support. Hollow out your abdomen to create length from your pubic bone to your navel—long and luscious—and stretch your lower back. After you curl down, sit up again—roll to your right side and then use your hands to help you up safely.

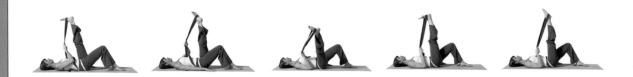

HAMSTRING, ANKLE, AND FOOT STRETCHES

Your hamstrings are a group of three posterior muscles that work together to flex your knees and extend your thighs. Collectively, your hamstrings are very long—attaching around your butt-bones, spanning down the back of your legs, and attaching in various positions around the back of your knees to perform slightly different functions. The biceps femoris is located on the outer back portion of the thigh and helps externally rotate your hips; the semitendinosis and semimembranosis are located on the inner back thigh and help internally rotate your hips.

To create harmony and length in the back of your legs and improve hip and joint mobility, you will stretch these muscles as a group. You may also find that stretching them will reduce stiffness and pain in your low back. When your hamstrings are chronically tight, you may experience back issues. For example, tight hamstrings can eventually affect the position of your pelvis. If this should happen, the natural arch of your low back will flatten, which may cause a change in your body position and create more serious problems, including pain radiating down your legs from compressed nerves and discs. Stretching can be your first line of defense.

HEAD TO TOE ALIGNMENT TIPS

✳

1. To lengthen and stretch your hamstrings correctly, you must align your pelvis. Make sure your hip bones are even. You can use your hands to push your hip bones into place. Aligning your pelvis properly is the only way to ensure that you're lengthening your hamstrings correctly.

2. Your sacrum should touch the floor.

3. Please pay attention to your neck and shoulders. If your chin is lifted to the ceiling, then you might have shoulder or neck tightness. Place a small pad or hand towel under your head so you can realign your head and neck. Don't work with a severe arch in your neck, which can injure delicate muscles, soft tissues, and cervical bones.

4. If you have a hamstring or groin injury, proceed very cautiously, if at all.

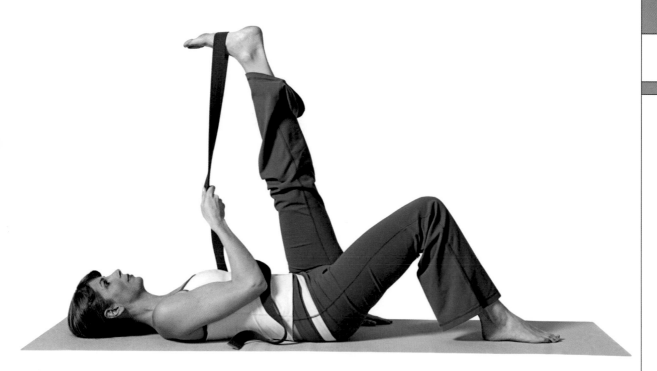

FUSING MIND AND MOTION

✳

Breathe continuously.
Each exhale will deepen your
stretch and create length in
your hamstrings.

1 Lie on your back with your knees bent, feet hip-width apart. Pull your left knee to your chest and wrap a towel or belt around the sole of your foot, making sure it's long enough so your head rests even on the floor, not jutting your chin to the ceiling. Straighten your left leg so your toes lengthen to the ceiling. Turn your toes out slightly. (If you can straighten your left leg, then straighten your right leg, firmly gluing the back of your thigh to the floor. If you can't straighten your left leg, keep your right knee bent.) Inhale for inspiration, then, as you exhale, slowly bring your toes toward your nose. Continue to press the back of your right thigh into the floor to stretch the front of that thigh. As you breathe, scoop your navel to your spine on each exhale, bringing your left leg closer to your nose. Complete three to five breaths and then continue stretching.

continued on next page ➤

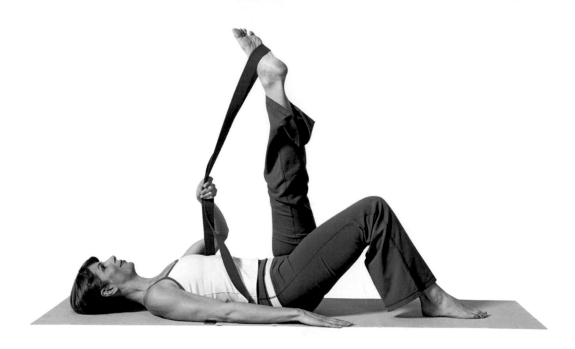

2 Use the belt to guide your left leg across the mid-line of your body, toes out slightly to stretch the outer hamstring and hip. As you breathe, focus on each exhale to ease tight hips. Complete three to five breaths and then continue stretching.

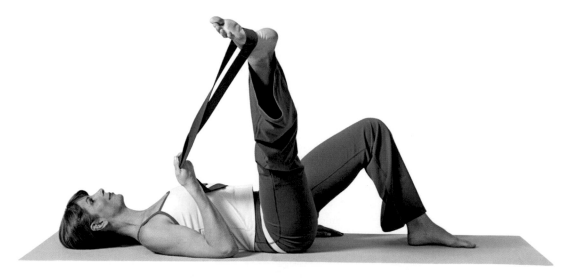

3 Use the strap to gently guide your left leg out away from your body. Relax your foot and focus on deepening your stretch while maintaining the correct alignment of your pelvis. You should feel a deep inner hip (groin) stretch, which includes your internal hamstrings. Complete three to five breaths and then switch legs.

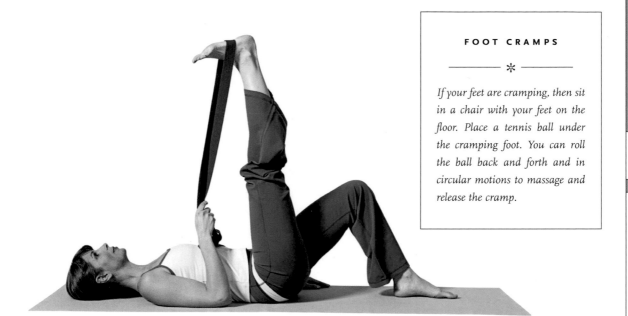

FOOT CRAMPS

———— ✳ ————

If your feet are cramping, then sit in a chair with your feet on the floor. Place a tennis ball under the cramping foot. You can roll the ball back and forth and in circular motions to massage and release the cramp.

4 After stretching your hamstrings, do three ankle rolls in and then reverse direction for three more. These ankle rolls will warm-up your ankle joints, increase your flexibility, and stretch your lower leg muscles. Finish this series by stretching your toes. Flex your foot by pushing your heel away from your face.

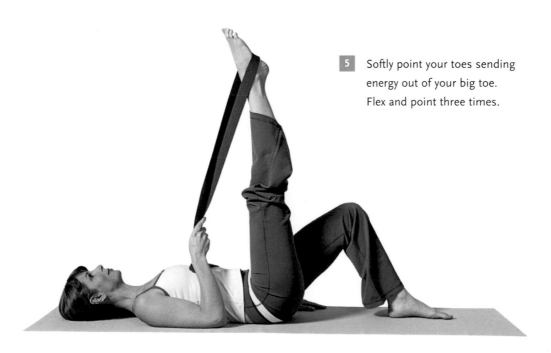

5 Softly point your toes sending energy out of your big toe. Flex and point three times.

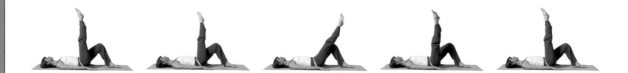

LEG CIRCLES

After the previous stretch, which is a nice warm up for your legs, you will perform Leg Circles. Besides increasing circulation in your hips and joints, this exercise will strengthen and shape areas of your body that can be very stubborn to tone—abs, thighs, and hips. Keep in mind that as the leg makes a circle, it should challenge your abdominals to stay centered!

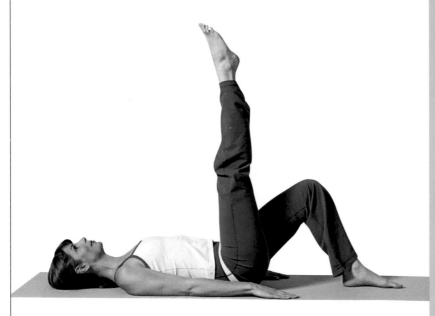

1 Lie on your back with your knees bent, feet hip-width apart. Use your hands to move your right knee to your chest and then stretch your leg to the ceiling and relax your toes. Next lengthen your arms by your side, palms down. Reach your toes long to the ceiling and slightly turn your foot out. As you inhale, bring your toes closer to your nose as your leg initiates the leg circle.

HEAD TO TOE ALIGNMENT TIPS

✳

1. Your pelvis must remain stable, no rocking from side to side, even though your leg will challenge your trunk stability. If you feel like you can't control this rocking, try pressing the palms of your hands and the back of your arms into the mat while melting each bone of your spine into the floor to help establish trunk stability. It's also very important that you exhale to engage your deep abdominals to help support your trunk and strengthen your abs.

2. Imagine a string tugging on your big toe, lifting it to the ceiling. Your leg should lengthen from your center and be as straight as possible.

3. Take every opportunity to contract your inner thighs, especially when your leg crosses your body.

FUSING MIND AND MOTION

✳

Inhale to send your breath into your lateral ribs.

✳✳✳

Breathe continuously as if the motion of your of leg and breath are one. Focus on exhaling as the leg circles to activate your transverse for trunk stability.

✳✳✳

Inhale to bring to your toes closer to your nose as your leg initiates the circle.

✳✳✳

Exhale to move your leg across your body, contracting your inner thighs.

✳✳✳

Continue exhaling to move your leg toward your heel and around up to your nose.

✳✳✳

Inhale to pause slightly before circling the leg again.

✳✳✳

Repeat five leg circles and then reverse the direction of the leg circles for five more.

✳✳✳

Switch legs.

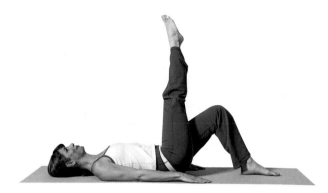

2 Exhale to move your leg across your body—imagine that your inner thighs kiss.

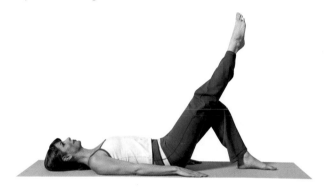

3 Continue to exhale and circle your leg to your heel.

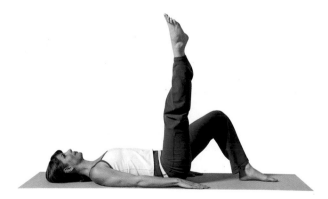

4 Continue to exhale and circle your leg to the side and then toward your nose. Inhale, pause for a second, and then circle the leg again. Your leg is active and straight as a needle! Scoop your belly to your spine with every circle.

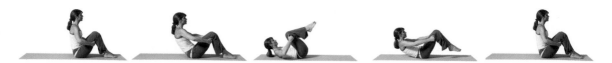

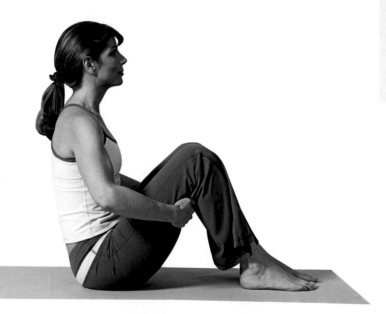

BABY ROCKING

This exercise will ease spinal tension, improve spinal flexibility, stretch the muscles of your back, send awareness to your abdominals by pulling your navel to your spine, and challenge your balance and pelvic stability.

Your goal is to learn how to balance on your butt bones (which are the bones you sit on) while pulling your navel to your spine. Sometimes, rocking can be difficult, especially if your abdominals are weak and you have tightness in your lower back. As a result, you may pound your lower back into the floor. Be careful; you don't want to strain your lower back.

FUSING MIND AND MOTION

✳

Your breath flows as the motion does, rocking back and forth.

✳✳✳

Inhale as you rock back.

✳✳✳

Exhale to rock forward, scooping your navel to protect your lower back.

✳✳✳

Repeat eight to ten times.

1 Sit on your bottom with your heels close to your butt bones, soles of your feet touching the floor. Place the palms of your hands behind your thighs.

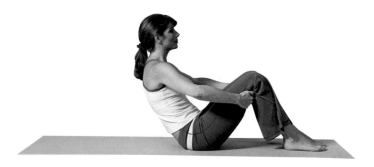

2 Practice a 6–12 curl, scooping your pubic bone up and navel in toward your spine as you exhale, hollowing your abdomen. Repeat three to five times.

When you feel in control, roll backward and balance on your tailbone.

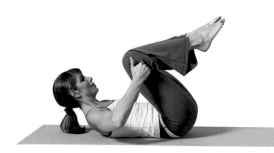

3 Continue to roll back until most of your body weight is on your mid back.

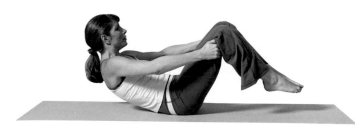

4 Gaze between your thighs as you rock forward and back, from your tailbone to your mid-back, scooping the entire time. Your head should never touch the mat.

HEAD TO TOE ALIGNMENT TIPS

❋

1. Rocking looks easy, but it can be a difficult exercise, especially if you have a combination of weak abdominals and lower back tightness. If you hear a "clunk-clunk" in your low back, then that's a sign that your lower back muscles are tight. Take it easy. If necessary, just lie on your back and pull your knees to your chest to relax tight back muscles. Also, you don't have to rock—just follow the before-rocking pictures to ease into this exercise.

2. While you're in this position, your shoulders may creep toward your ears. Watch out—this creates unnecessary tension and stress in your entire spine, especially in your head, neck, and shoulders. Let it go—ease your tension.

SINGLE LEG STRETCH (WALL)

This exercise will strengthen your abdominals, coordinate your breath with your movement, teach you how to stabilize your trunk while your arm and legs challenge it, and increase your coordination and concentration.

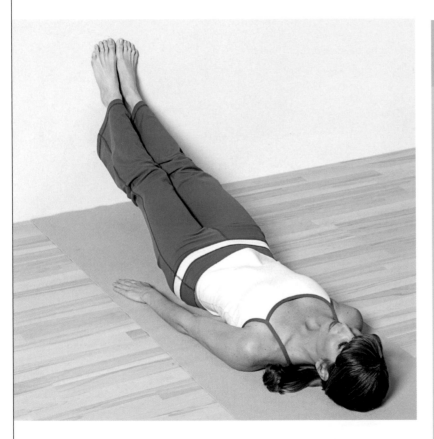

1 Lie on your back with your legs extended and walk your feet up the wall so your toes are in line with your nose. Arms lengthen by your sides.

HEAD TO TOE ALIGNMENT TIPS

✳

1. If you have a neck injury, don't do this exercise.

2. Even in these early stages, imagine your leg stretching for miles as your big toe lengthens away from your hips.

3. If your neck tires, rest your head at any point or work with a pillow under your head.

4. Maintain a stable spine even though your legs are moving and challenging its stability.

5. Don't look up at the ceiling, rather gaze between your thighs.

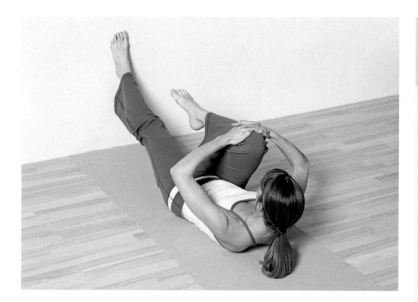

2 Use your right hand to bring your right knee to your chest. Interlace your fingers on your knee. Curl your chin to your chest so the back of your shoulders come off the mat and gaze between your thighs. Inhale to give your right knee a little hug, pulling it closer to your chest with a second pulse.

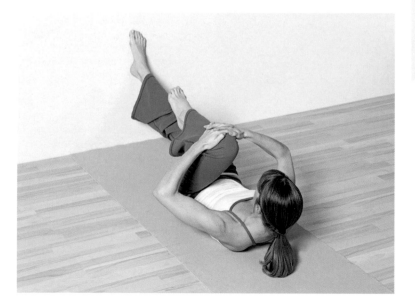

3 Continue inhaling as you switch legs, pulling your left knee to your chest with your interlaced hands while placing your right foot on the wall. Then, as you exhale, repeat the same leg directions, switching legs each time.

FUSING MIND AND MOTION

✳

Inhale gradually, bringing your right knee to your chest with a slight pulse while lengthening your left foot toward the wall. Switch legs so your left knee moves toward your chest and your right foot lengthens to the wall.

✳✳✳

Exhale gradually, bringing your right knee to your chest with a slight pulse while extending your left foot to the wall. Switch legs, so the left knee moves toward your chest and the right foot lengthens to the wall. This entire cycle totals one set of leg stretches.

✳✳✳

Repeat four sets.

DOUBLE LEG STRETCH (WALL)

After completing Single Leg Stretch, move quickly into Double Leg Stretch. This exercise will also challenge your trunk stability, strengthen your abdominals, and increase your coordination and concentration. Continue to focus on your neck. If you feel any tension, lower your head to the floor to rest before proceeding with this exercise.

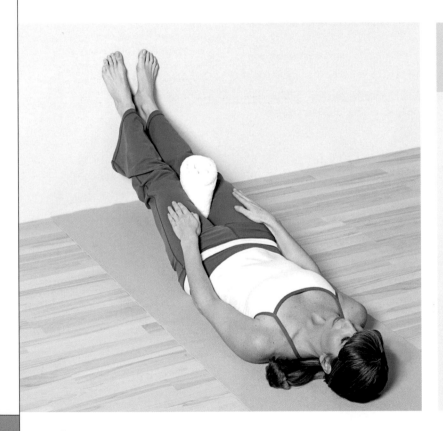

FUSING MIND AND MOTION

✳

Your breath will flow as your arms challenge your core.

* * *

Inhale your arms over your head, fingers reaching toward the ceiling.

* * *

Exhale your arms to your thighs, scooping your belly to protect your lower back.

* * *

Repeat four to eight times.

1 Lie on your back with your legs extended and walk your feet up the wall so your toes are in line with your nose. Place a rolled up towel between your thighs and then rest your hands on top of your thighs.

1. Don't do this exercise if you have a neck injury.

2. Don't forget to squeeze the towel to feel the pelvic floor engagement.

3. If you neck tires, you can rest it any time during this work or place a pillow under your head for support—no straining.

4. Remember correct spinal alignment—neck long as your chin moves toward your chest, eyes gazing between your legs.

5. Melt your spine into the mat as your arms lift and lower and challenge your trunk stability.

6. As your arms lift over your head, your ribs may lift as well. Pay attention to your rib placement. Remember ribs close to your hips to engage your abdominals, specifically your obliques.

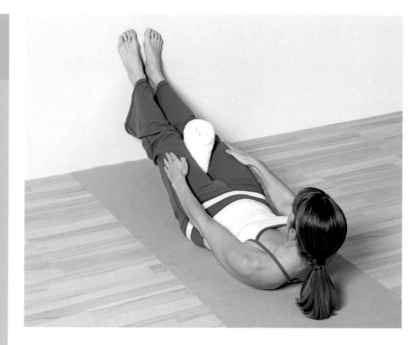

2 With a stable trunk and pelvis, lift your head so your eyes gaze between your thighs.

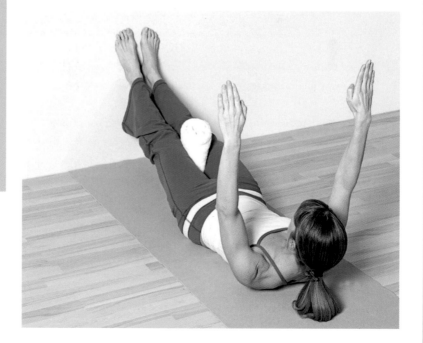

3 Inhale to lift your arms over your head, fingertips reaching toward the ceiling. Then, as you exhale, lower them to your thighs.

PRONE BREATHING

This exercise will stretch your lower spine, improve spinal flexibility, send awareness to your pelvis area, challenge your Pilates breath in a face down position, increase your breathing capacity, and strengthen your abdominals. Your goals are to engage your deep stabilizing muscles: transverse, multifidus, and pelvic floors. Despite your belly being supported by the floor, try to lift the pit of your belly up to your spine.

HEAD TO TOE ALIGNMENT TIPS

✳

1. Relax and focus on your Pilates breath.

2. Don't elevate your shoulders as you breathe in, rather grow from within to open each rib.

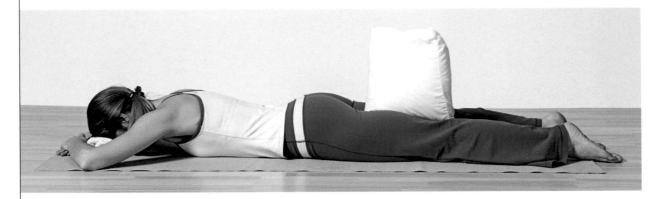

1 Lie face down and extend your legs. Place a small pillow between your inner thighs and rest your forehead on a small towel.

2 Cross your hands overhead and just relax. Inhale deeply, sending your breath into your lateral ribs, which may flare your back slightly. Exhale to gently lift the pit of your belly to your spine while you maintain a neutral and stable pelvis. As you lengthen your exhalation, your lumbar spine will extend and stretch.

FUSING MIND AND MOTION

✳

Inhale to expand your ribs laterally, opening each separate rib if you can.

✳ ✳ ✳

Exhale to pull your belly button to your spine and stretch and lengthen your lower back.

✳ ✳ ✳

Repeat this movement five times, but feel free to do as many as you want—it's such a yummy stretch for your lower back.

PILLOW SQUEEZE (PRONE)

This exercise will strengthen your abdominals, pelvic floors, and inner thighs; ease spinal tension; and send awareness to your pelvic floors.

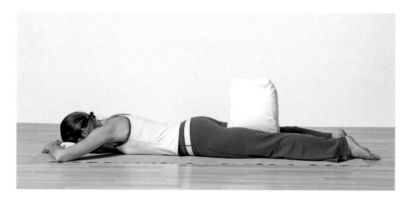

1 Lie face down with your legs extended. Place a small pillow between your legs and rest your forehead on a small towel. Cross your hands overhead to relax. Inhale deeply to send your breath into your lateral ribs until you feel the ribs opening.

FUSING MIND AND MOTION

*

Inhale to expand and open each rib in your back.

* * *

Exhale and squeeze the pillow to feel the inner pull coming deep within your pelvis.

* * *

Repeat five to eight times.

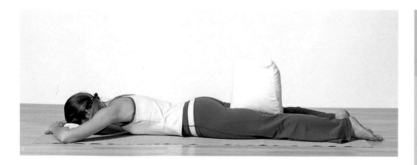

2 As you exhale, lift your belly button to your spine and squeeze the pillow between your legs to feel the muscles between your legs contract. Maintain a stable pelvis, even as your belly button pulls up to the spine. Don't engage your hamstrings or any other buttocks muscles. This contraction comes from deep within your pelvic floor muscles.

HEAD TO TOE ALIGNMENT TIPS

*

1. Don't move your pelvis. The idea is to contract between your thighs and engage your pelvic floor muscles without creating any tension for your lower back—it's a deep inner pull upward, like a Kegel exercise.

2. Relax your upper body. Again, the only part of your body working is the area of muscles between your inner thighs.

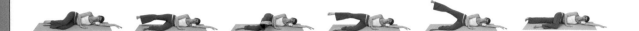

PILATES LITE

LEG WORK

These leg exercises will tighten and tone your inner and outer thighs, ease tension in your hips, challenge your trunk stability in a sideline position, and lengthen your legs. Of course, proper alignment is vital to strengthening your body correctly, so let's begin with proper alignment for all sideline leg exercises: hips are stacked on one another; shoulders are square; and your head, neck, and shoulders are relaxed.

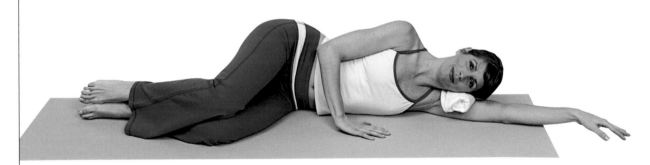

1 Lie on your left side with your back flat against a wall. Bend your knees and stack them directly on top of one another, which will also align your hip bones. Reach your left arm out straight above your head and place a small hand towel between your ear and the top of your arm.

FUSING MIND AND MOTION

*

If the breathing instructions are too difficult to follow, then just breathe normally, making sure you don't hold your breath.

* * *

Repeat each exercise eight to ten times and then switch legs.

HEAD TO TOE
ALIGNMENT TIPS

✳

1. Try anchoring your back to the wall to help keep your trunk stable—eventually you will be able to support your own trunk and won't need the wall's support.

2. Your hip bones should be even and stacked on top of one another. You might want to take your hand and push your hip bones into place, making sure they are even before you begin moving your legs.

3. Relax your head, neck, and shoulders.

4. Remember the goal is to work your outer and inner thighs, not your waist, so pay attention to the alignment of your hip bones. Don't let your hips lift toward your shoulders.

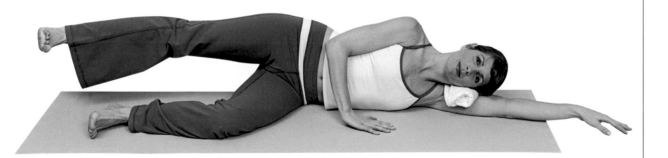

2 Straighten your right leg and flex your foot. Hold this position for three to five breaths.

continued on next page ➤

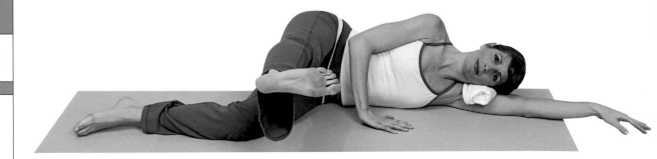

3 Inhale to move your leg forward. Your back should remain in contact with the wall. Your hip bones are stacked.

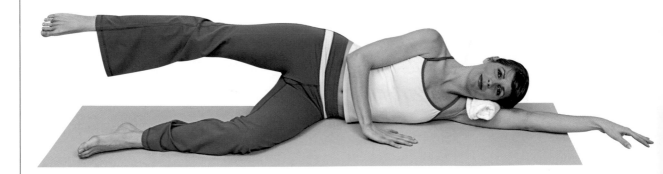

4 Exhale to move your leg back to the wall, contracting your glutes. After completing five to eight sets, return your leg to the starting position.

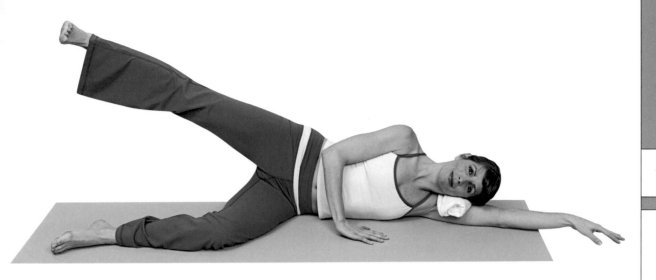

5 Inhale to lift your leg toward the ceiling, knee facing front to tighten and tone your outer thighs. Exhale to lower your leg. If you would like to add a little resistance, place your hand on your outer thigh and press down as you lift your leg. After completing five to eight sets, return to the starting position.

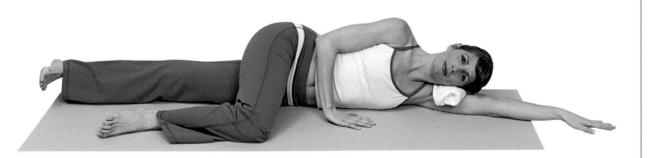

6 Move your right leg and bend it over your left leg. Rest your right knee on the floor with your thigh at a 90-degree angle. Straighten your left leg. Breathe naturally as you lift your left leg off the floor about an inch or two. Hold this position as you lengthen your leg away from your center. This lift comes from your center and inner thighs. If you need more of a challenge, add eight to ten pulses to strengthen your inner thighs.

CHILD'S POSE

Here's your treat: Child's Pose. This stretch will ease tension in your back, relieve any lower back strain from this workout, and soothe any frazzled nerves.

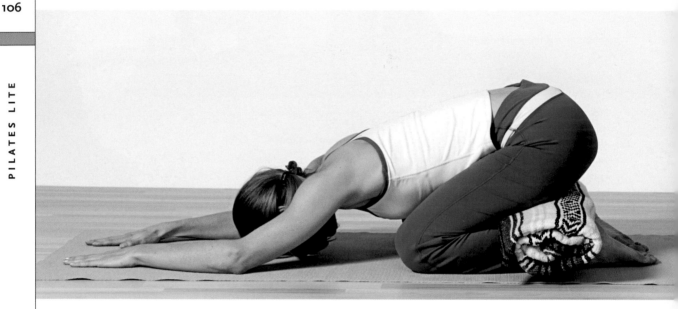

1 From the face down position, sit back so your bottom rests on your heels. You might need to open your knees wider to drop your bottom to your heels. If you can't sit back on your heels, then place a blanket underneath your buttocks for support. At the same time, reach your arms out in front to stretch your upper back and shoulder muscles. Breathe and just relax. Congratulations, you're done!

STRETCHING YOUR LIMITS

✳

Congratulations, you have just completed level one! When you feel confident that you can perform all of these exercises with correct alignment and without stressing your body, then you can move on to level two. Remember, stable and scoop! Below are some chapter highlights:

* * *

Here's where it all begins: total concentration, control of movement, centering your body, and connecting with your breath.

* * *

Each exercise in this chapter simulates classic Pilates exercises while focusing on the fundamentals so you gain more strength, flexibility, and awareness in your own body.

* * *

If your belly bulges at any point, then you're no longer working your transverse. The rectus abdominus (the most superficial muscle) has taken over, which might result in a permanent bulge if you keep training with poor form— no loaf of bread in the belly!

* * *

Focus on stabilizing your spine and scooping your belly button to your navel, hugging your abs to your spine the whole time. Stable and scoop.

* * *

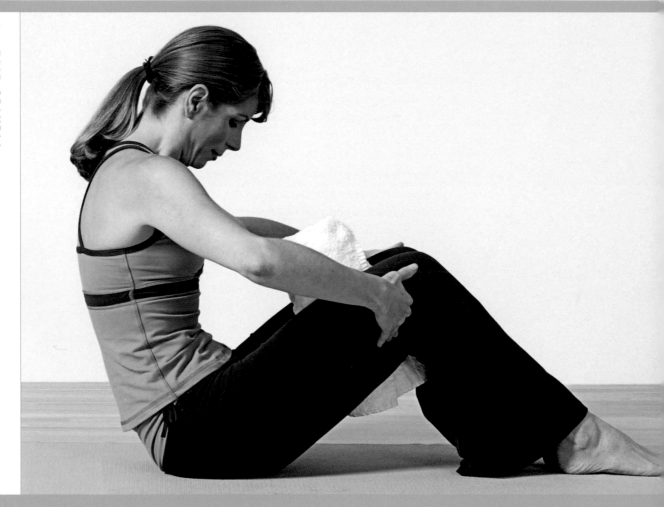

CHAPTER FIVE

ONE MUSCLE AT A TIME

PERHAPS WHILE GOING THROUGH YOUR DAY, you have had a moment to wonder how you do it. Daily life requires you to have plenty of functional strength—when you hail a cab, walk the dog, or ski a slope. In this chapter, you will continue to build more strength, balance, mobility, and coordination—all important aspects of (what else?) functional fitness!

What is functional fitness? It's a current trend of training that combines strength, balance, coordination, and stability challenges that simulate the same motions you do in your everyday life. When it comes to functional, you don't have to bulk uplike a body builder, rather you need useful strength so you are ready for whatever life throws your way. Simply put, Pilates defines functional.

THE PLAN

By now, you have built some muscle and mental memory, which is good, because this next set of exercises builds on what you have already done, but requires more from you. More balance! More strength! More coordination! Try to do this workout three to four times a week for about six weeks before advancing to the Classic Pilates mat work in the next chapter. Below is a review of what you learned in the last chapter:

* You've mastered the 60-second body scan. You should be able to feel the difference between good alignment and bad alignment.

* You've worked on keeping your trunk stable, especially your pelvis, and you've scooped your navel to your spine at all times.

* You've focused on your breathing: You're getting better at directing your inhalation into your back ribs and lengthening your exhale.

YOUR GOALS FOR CHAPTER FIVE:

level two

* Deepen your Pilates breath so you can increase your breathing capacity and strengthen your stabilizing muscles. Centering will now be more difficult as the intensity of the exercises increases.

* Focus on the inner pull through your pelvic floors. You will work with a small hand towel or pillow between your thighs to reinforce this contraction.

* Move with control—absolutely no haphazard movements.

* Concentrate on scooping your abdominals, stabilizing your trunk, and now squeezing your inner thighs—stable, scoop, and squeeze.

* Look in the mirror because you should see some visible results!

SEQUENCE OF EXERCISES
*ONE MUSCLE
AT A TIME*

✳

THE FIFTY
(WITH TOWEL)

ROLL UP (MODIFIED)

HAMSTRING STRETCH
(CHAPTER 4)

LEG CIRCLES

ROLLING LIKE A BALL
(MODIFIED)

SINGLE LEG STRETCH

DOUBLE LEG STRETCH

CAT TO SEXY CAT

FLIGHT

LEG WORK
Side Kicks
Heel Beats
Inner Thigh Circles

SEAL

THE FIFTY
(WITH TOWEL)

This exercise will strengthen your abdominals, warm up your body, increase your breathing capacity, and improve your coordination. This next level takes your feet off the wall, so centering will require a great deal of abdominal strength plus coordination— your goal is to center and hold your legs in position while pumping your arms, without any movement or bouncing in your torso.

Place a towel between your thighs to strengthen your inner thighs and pelvic floors while sending awareness to that area to concentrate on the inner lift. The breathing is exactly the same as in the earlier version of the exercise.

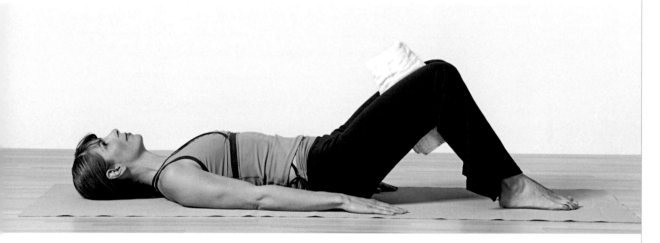

1 Lie on your back with your knees bent, feet hip-width apart. Place a towel between your knees. Lengthen your arms by your sides, palms down.

continued on next page ➤

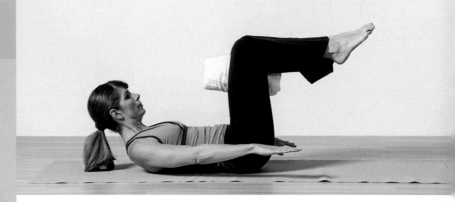

HEAD TO TOE ALIGNMENT TIPS

❋

1. If you have or have had a neck injury, please talk to your doctor before doing this exercise. If your neck tires before your body, then reevaluate how you're holding your head. Your head is an extension of your neck, so think long even as you curl your chin to your chest.

2. Don't bounce your trunk as your arms pump up and down. Center your middle so no other body part moves except your arms.

3. Squeeze the pillow to engage your pelvic floors.

4. If you feel any lower back strain, lift your toes so they are above your knees or higher. If your back strain continues, place your feet on the wall.

5. If you experience any new sensations, such as pangs, pops, or twinges, stop immediately.

2 Lift your knees to your chest so they are in a 90-degree angle with your hips (knees directly over hip bones). Curl your chin to your chest and lift the back of your shoulders off the floor—lengthen your neck while lifting the palms of your hands off the floor about two inches. Stretch your fingertips long. Inhale to pump your arms up and down vigorously for a count of five, then, as you exhale, pump your arms for a count of five—creating resistance in the length of your arms, like you are pushing against something.

FUSING MIND AND MOTION

❋

Pump your arms about six to eight inches.

✳ ✳ ✳

Inhale for five counts and exhale for five counts.

✳ ✳ ✳

Repeat five breath cycles.

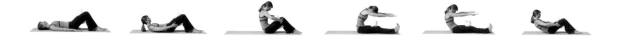

ROLL UP (MODIFIED)

This exercise will strengthen your abdominal muscles, send awareness to your spine, and increase spinal flexibility. This is your first exercise to move you through full spinal articulation, meaning every bone of your spine will touch the mat—imagine peeling your spine off the mat as if lifting a strand of pearls.

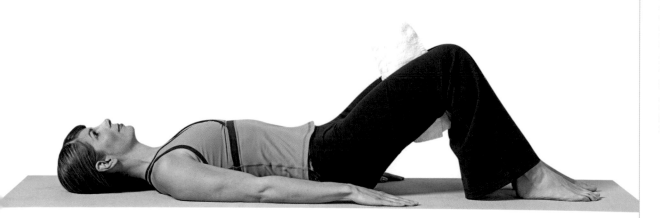

1 Lie on your back with your knees bent, feet hip-width apart. Place a rolled-up towel between your thighs. Lengthen your arms by your sides.

continued on next page ➤

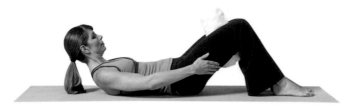

2 Wrap your hands around your thighs, then inhale to curl your chin to your chest—neck long.

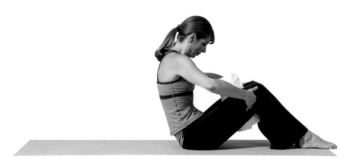

3 Exhale to lift your shoulders off the ground and roll up; hollow your belly and squeeze the towel at the same time. Use your hands to help you curl up so you don't jump or jerk up.

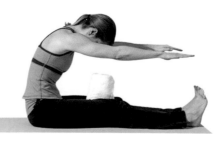

4 Continue to exhale and straighten your legs while reaching your fingertips past your toes.

HEAD TO TOE ALIGNMENT TIPS

✳

1. Relax your jaw, mouth, neck, and shoulders— no tensing during this motion.

2. Move within control, no jerking your body through any motion, which may strain your lower back. If you can't roll up with control, use your hands to guide you up and lower you down.

3. Don't straighten your torso or lift your front ribs— remember scoop and curl, scoop and curl. Your spine stays rounded as you roll up and roll down. Gaze at your belly button to remind you to stay rounded and relax your head, neck, and shoulders.

4. If you do this exercise correctly, in addition to strength, you will gain long abdominals. Focus on curling up, not crunching. While curling down, focus on lengthening your abdominals from your pubic bone to the bottom of your breastbone as every bone touches the mat. Imagine long and luscious abs!

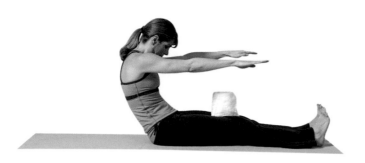

5 Inhale to tip your pubic bone to the ceiling, initiating the curl down.

**FUSING MIND
AND MOTION**

✻

Inhale to curl your chin to your
chest, gazing at your toes.

* * *

Exhale to lift your shoulders off
the floor and round over.

* * *

Inhale to initiate the curl down.

* * *

Exhale to lower your spine to the
mat, bone by bone.

* * *

Repeat three to five times.

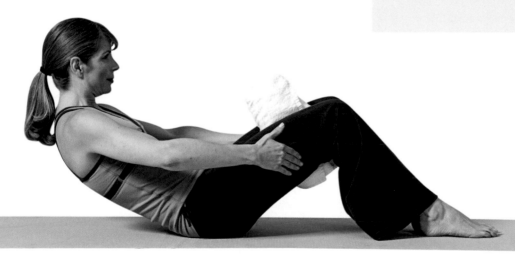

6 As you exhale, bend your knees and squeeze the pillow to scoop your
belly as you curl down bone by bone. Each bone of your spine will
touch the mat. Use your hands to guide your torso to the floor so
you don't just plop down.

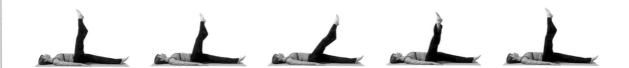

LEG CIRCLES

This exercise will warm up your hips, tighten and tone your hips and thighs, strengthen your abdominals, and nourish your hip joints. In this level, both legs will be straight, but the movement is still small as you draw a circle on the ceiling. The goal is to challenge your abdominals to keep your hips bones even and your pelvis stable in the movement. Imagine your leg circling like a pendulum in your hip socket while your hips remain stable.

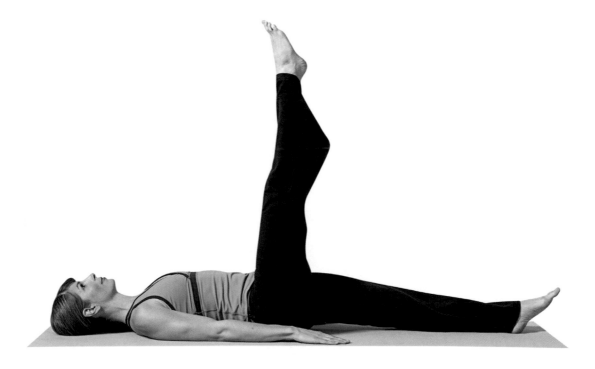

1 Lie on your back with your legs extended and neck long. Lengthen your arms by your sides, palms down. Move your right knee to your chest and then straighten your leg, toes turned out slightly. Relax your foot or softly point your toes. While your right leg is active, your left leg firmly presses into the floor—imagine the letter "L." Inhale to move your leg toward your nose.

**FUSING MIND
AND MOTION**

✳

Flow your breath with
each leg circle.

* * *

Inhale to move your leg
toward your nose.

* * *

Exhale to draw a circle on
the ceiling with your toes:
your leg crosses the midline
of your body, down to the
opposite foot, and circles
around to stop at your nose,
contracting your inner thighs
the whole time.

* * *

Repeat five leg circles and
then reverse the circle for five.
Then switch to opposite leg.

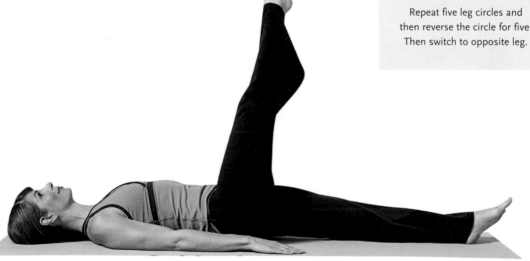

2 Exhale to move your right leg across your body; inner thighs squeeze.

continued on next page ➤

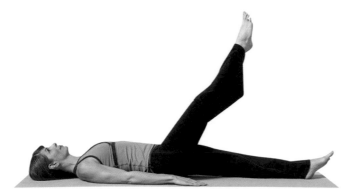

3 Continue to exhale while moving your leg to the opposite foot.

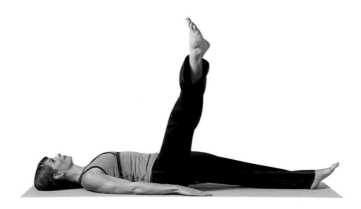

4 Continue to exhale and circle your leg to the side and up toward your nose. Inhale, pause slightly, then circle your leg again. Do a total of five circles and then reverse for five.

HEAD TO TOE ALIGNMENT TIPS

※

1. Don't rock your hips from side to side as you circle your leg. Keep the circles small at first.

2. Stabilize your trunk. If you feel centering is difficult, try pressing the palms of your hands, back of your arms, and the back of your head firmly into the mat to help stabilize your trunk while your leg challenges it.

3. Don't forget to drag out your exhale, which will also assist in pulling your belly button to your spine to help strengthen and stabilize your middle muscles.

4. Imagine a string pulling your big toe to the ceiling to lengthen your leg.

5. Before Leg Circles, stretch your hamstrings. Turn to page 92 in chapter 4 for a review, if necessary.

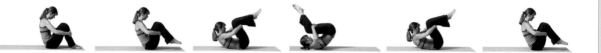

ROLLING LIKE A BALL (MODIFIED)

Rolling Like a Ball will ease spinal tension, stretch your spine, challenge your abdominals, and improve your balance. Focus on your abdominals—as you gain abdominal strength and are able to pull your abdominal wall closer to your spine, you should also feel a nice lower back stretch.

FUSING MIND AND MOTION

✳

Your breath flows as the roll does.

✳✳✳

Inhale to roll back.

✳✳✳

Exhale to roll up, scooping your navel in and up to protect your lower back.

✳✳✳

Repeat six to ten times.

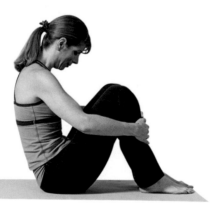

1 Sit on your bottom with your heels close, feet on the floor. Place the palms of your hands around your shins and stretch your elbows out to your sides. Open your knees wide. Lower your head so you gaze at your belly. Practice scooping your belly to warm up your spine.

continued on next page ➤

2 After warming up, place your hands behind your thighs. Scoop your navel to your spine and lift your toes off the ground so they hover about two to three inches off the floor.

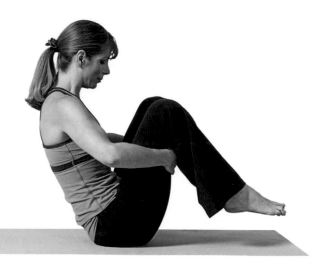

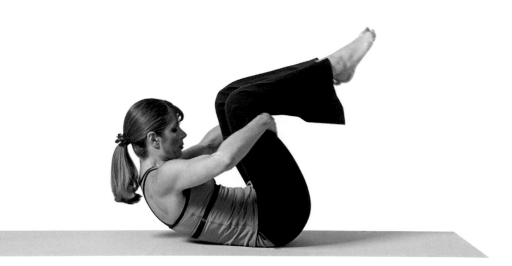

3 Inhale to roll back, eyes on your belly.

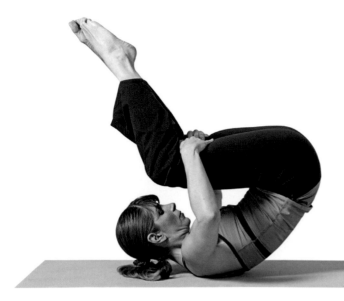

4 Continue to inhale and roll to your upper back. Your head never touches the mat. Exhale to roll up and balance on your tailbone so your toes hover off the floor to strengthen your belly muscles. After a few seconds, roll again, scooping your belly to control your pelvis.

HEAD TO TOE
ALIGNMENT TIPS

✳

1. Rolling seems easy, but it can be a difficult exercise, especially if your abdominals are weak or you have some lower back tightness. If you hear or feel a "clunk-clunk" in your lower back as you roll, stop rolling. This "clunk-clunk" usually indicates tightness in your lower back. Review Rocking in chapter 4, which stretches tight back muscles.

2. Don't lift your shoulders toward your ears as you roll. Relax your head, neck, jaw, and shoulders. This way, you won't create unnecessary tension and stress in your upper spine.

3. Don't throw your head back when you roll. Always look at your belly. Remember your head is an extension of your spine, so treat it well.

4. Stay curved in your torso, rounding over, yet pulling your belly button up and in to engage your abdominal muscles for support.

5. And finally, if you can't control the roll and feel very wobbly in your pelvis, try scooping deeper. Also, it is okay if your toes touch the floor for a split second if you need help balancing. But take every opportunity to balance, because that is the goal of this exercise, in addition to establishing multi-muscle control and strength.

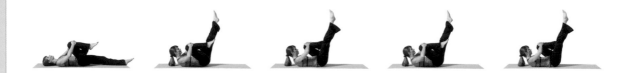

SINGLE LEG STRETCH

Single Leg Stretch will strengthen your abdominals as you focus on stabilizing your trunk against the movement of your arms and legs, challenge your leg and arm coordination, tone your hips and thighs, improve your concentration, and encourage you to flow your limbs from your center.

HEAD TO TOE ALIGNMENT TIPS

✳

1. If you have a neck injury, don't do this exercise.

2. Even in these early stages, imagine your leg stretching for miles as the big toe lengthens away from your hips.

3. Contract your bottom to tone your butt and thighs as you lengthen your leg away from your center.

4. Maintain trunk stability even though your legs are challenging it.

5. Don't look up at the ceiling; gaze between your thighs.

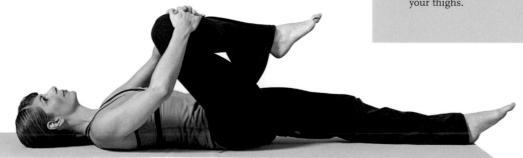

1 Lie on your back with your legs straight. Interlace your fingers and place your hands on your right knee and pull it toward your chest.

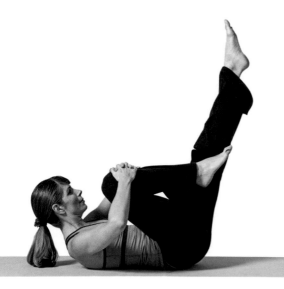

FUSING MIND AND MOTION

✼

Inhale gradually, bringing your right knee to your chest with a slight pulse while lengthening your left foot toward the ceiling. Switch legs so your left knee moves toward your chest and your right foot lengthens to the ceiling.

* * *

Exhale gradually, bringing your right knee to your chest with a slight pulse while extending your left foot to the ceiling. Switch legs, so the left knee moves toward your chest and the right foot lengthens to the ceiling— force all the air out of your lungs to flatten your belly. This entire cycle totals one set of leg stretches.

* * *

Repeat four sets.

2 As you inhale, curl your chin to your chest so your shoulders lift off the floor. Gaze between your thighs and give your right knee a little hug, pulling it closer to your chest. At the same time, lengthen your left leg to the ceiling, reaching long with your toes.

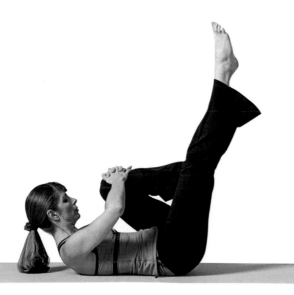

3 Continue inhaling and switch legs, moving your interlaced hands to pull your left knee to your chest while lengthening your right foot to the ceiling. Then, as you exhale, repeat.

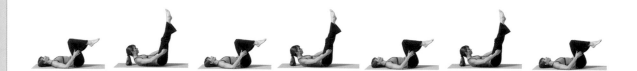

DOUBLE LEG STRETCH

Double Leg Stretch will strengthen your abdominals, improve your coordination, challenge your trunk stability against the movement of your legs, send awareness to your pelvic floors and inner thighs, and teach you how to flow your limbs from your center. You can work with a towel between your thighs to help stabilize your legs while you move them.

FUSING MIND AND MOTION

✳

Inhale to lengthen your legs to the ceiling.

✳✳✳

Exhale to lower your legs to your chest, emptying your lungs completely.

✳✳✳

Repeat four to eight times.

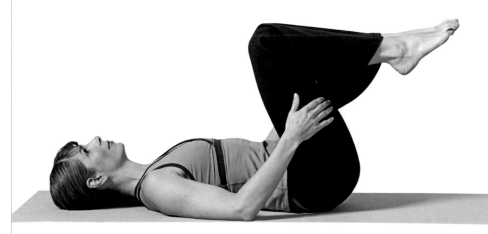

1   Lie on your back with your knees bent. Wrap your hands around your thighs.

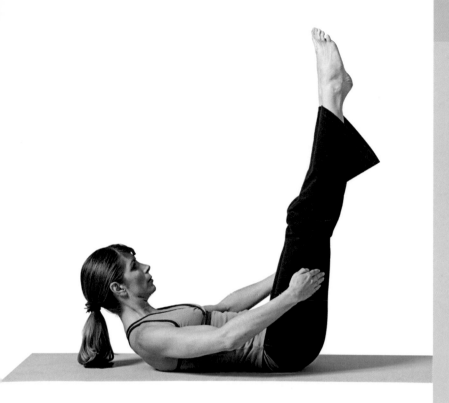

HEAD TO TOE ALIGNMENT TIPS

❋

1. Don't do this exercise if you have a neck injury.

2. Imagine stretching your legs for miles as your toes lengthen away from your hips.

3. Squeeze to engage your inner thighs and pelvic floors.

4. Don't look up at the ceiling. Your neck is long as you gaze between your thighs.

5. Melt every bone of your mid and lower spine into the mat, especially when your legs lengthen away from your center.

2 As you inhale, curl your chin to your chest to lift your shoulders off the mat and lengthen your legs to the ceiling. Exhale to lower your legs to your chest, but keep your head up and gaze between your thighs; lengthen your neck. Repeat four to eight times.

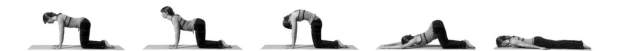

CAT TO SEXY CAT

This exercise will ease back tension (which is especially nice after Single and Double Leg Stretch), teach you how to activate your deep abdominals to stretch your spine, encourage a neutral spine position, and strengthen your abdominals.

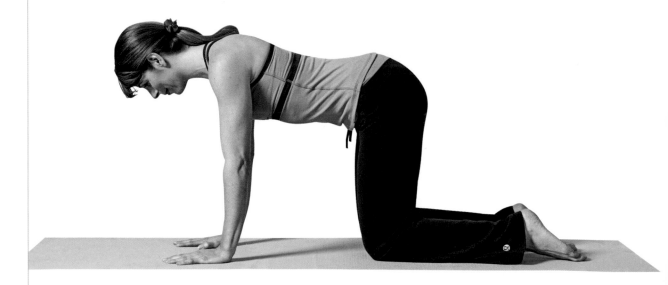

1 In a kneeling position, place your hands directly under your shoulders and your knees directly under your hip bones. Maintain a neutral spine by sliding your shoulder blades down your back and making sure your hip bones are even.

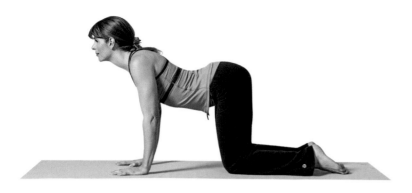

2 Inhale to drop your belly button to the floor, arching your back.

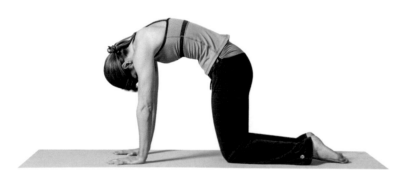

3 Exhale to pull your navel to your spine, engaging your deep abdominals to stretch the length of your spine. Imagine a cat stretching from the top of its head to its tailbone.

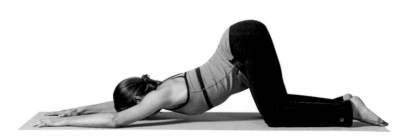

4 From cat, slide your belly along the floor while arching your back so you look like a sexy cat until you're lying on your belly. Relax.

FUSING MIND AND MOTION

✻

Inhale and drop your belly button to the floor.

✳ ✳ ✳

Exhale to round your back and stretch your spine.

✳ ✳ ✳

Repeat four to eight times and then slide to the floor like a sexy cat to get ready for Flight.

HEAD TO TOE ALIGNMENT TIPS

✻

1. If you have a lower back issues, please check with your doctor before arching your spine.

2. Even though this stretch feels oh-so-good, work with proper alignment or within your Pilates box, meaning your arms and legs don't extend past your shoulder and hip joints.

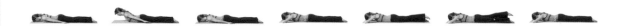

FLIGHT

This exercise will strengthen the muscles of your back, buttocks, and hamstrings; keep your spine healthy; heighten pelvis awareness; and challenge your shoulder blades to slide down your spine. Your goal is to develop a sense of where your pelvis and shoulder blades are while moving your limbs. You need to maintain a stable (neutral) spine even though you are in a face down position.

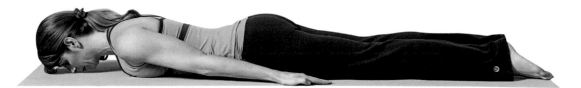

1 Lie on your stomach with your arms by your side, palms down.
Lift the pit of your belly up to your spine.

2 Inhale to slowly lift your chest off the floor, walking your fingertips toward your toes. Slide your shoulder blades down your back, engaging your upper back muscles. Next, lift your arms an inch or two and keep extending out through your fingertips. Exhale to lower your body and arms to the floor.

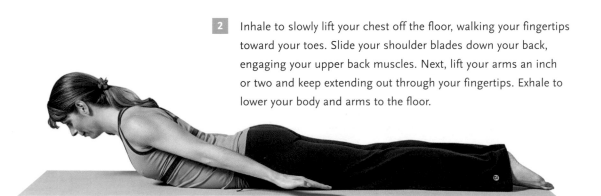

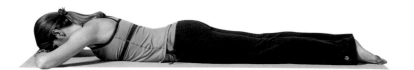

3 Lie on your stomach with your legs lengthened behind you. This time, place your arms over your head, crossing them at the wrist. Rest your forehead on your arms and relax your upper back.

FUSING MIND AND MOTION

✳

Inhale to lift and extend your body and limbs.

* * *

Exhale to gently lower to the floor.

* * *

Repeat three to five times.

HEAD TO TOE ALIGNMENT TIPS

✳

1. Don't push into your lower back. Relax your back.

2. When lifting your arms, don't elevate your shoulders to your ears. Keep reaching your fingertips toward your toes to slide your shoulder blades down your back to strengthen your upper body muscles in correct alignment.

3. When lifting your legs, engage your buttocks and hamstrings. Again, relax your back.

4. Watch and feel for increasing pressure in your lumbar spine as your legs lift. Your pelvis may shift forward due the increasing weight of your leg. Maintain a neutral and stable pelvis. If you can't, then don't lift the leg very high, especially if you feel any pressure in your lower back.

5. Don't flip your head back. Look at the floor to lengthen the muscles in the back of your neck.

6. Pay attention to your shoulders and pelvis—maintain a neutral position in both.

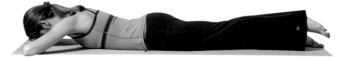

4 Inhale to lift your left leg about an inch off the ground. Pay attention to your pelvis—absolutely no movement! Exhale, gently placing your leg on the floor.

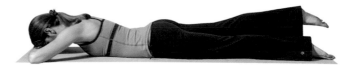

5 Inhale to lift your right leg about an inch off the ground. Pull your belly button to your spine to maintain your stable (neutral) pelvis position. Rest in Child's Pose.

LEG WORK
SIDE KICKS, HEEL BEATS, AND INNER THIGH CIRCLES

These leg exercises will tone and tighten your thighs, challenge your trunk stability while you're on your side, open your hips, nourish your hip joints, and encourage you to flow your legs from your center. At this level, you will increase the intensity of your leg work by taking your body off the wall. Get ready for a visible lower body transformation!

---

*

SIDE KICKS

This leg exercise will tone and tighten your thighs and buttocks, challenge your trunk stability, and open and stretch tight hips and hamstrings.

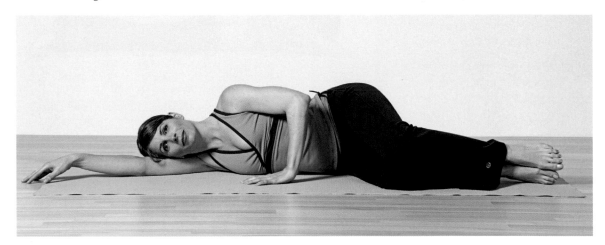

1 Lie on your right side with your legs bent. Align both hip bones so they are stacked on top of one another. Straighten your right arm and rest your head it. Your left arm reaches forward to support your torso; square your shoulders.

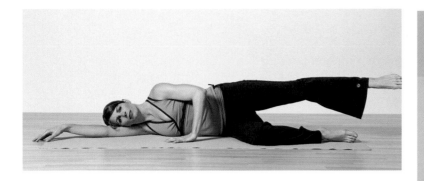

2 Lift and extend your left leg to hip-height. Hold this position for five breaths. Stop here if this is challenging for you.

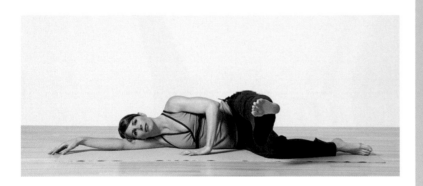

3 Inhale to swing your leg forward—maintain a stable pelvis and solid trunk.

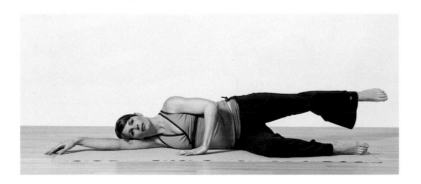

4 Exhale to swing your leg back to work your bottom.

ONE MUSCLE AT A TIME

HEAD TO TOE ALIGNMENT TIPS

*

1. As you swing your leg forward, its weight may roll your hip forward. Remember hips stay stacked on top of one another and scoop your belly to help stabilize your trunk.

2. As you swing your leg back, its weight may cause your ribs to lift and your back to arch. Pull your navel to your spine and drop your ribs to your hips to help activate all abdominal muscles.

3. Do six to eight sets then move on to the next exercise, Heel Beats.

HEEL BEATS

This leg exercise will tone and tighten your inner thighs,
challenge your trunk stability, and encourage you to contract
your pelvic floor muscles.

1 Lie on your right side with
your legs extended. Bend
your right leg so both hip
bones are stacked on top of
one another. Turn your left leg
up so your knee faces the
ceiling. Straighten your right
arm and rest your head on
top of it. Reach your left arm
forward to support your
torso. Inhale to lift your
left leg to the ceiling. Your
knee faces up as your toes
lengthen—imagine miles
and miles of leg.

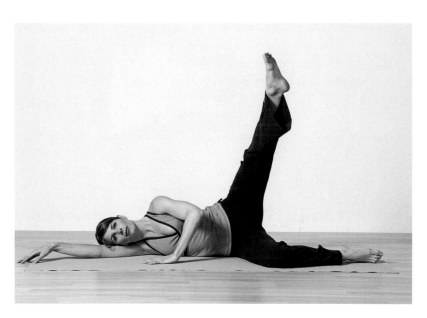

HEAD TO TOE
ALIGNMENT TIPS

✳

1. Maintain a stable center,
keeping your hips stacked.

2. As the top leg lowers to the
bottom, try to lengthen it
longer than the bottom leg.

3. Repeat six times and
then get ready for Inner
Thigh Circles.

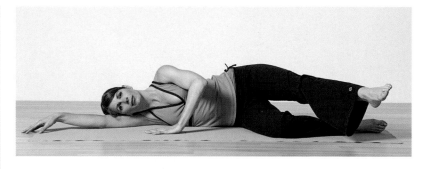

2 Exhale to lower the left leg to your right leg, leading with your heel
and contracting between your thighs. Count to four as you lower your
leg and engage your inner thighs.

INNER THIGH CIRCLES

This leg exercise will tone and tighten your inner thighs and encourage you to contract your pelvic floor muscles.

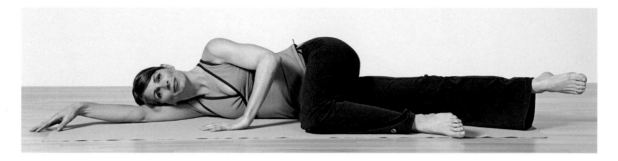

1 Cross your left leg over your right leg to rest your knee on the ground, leg bent at 90-degrees. Lift your right leg to begin leg circles.

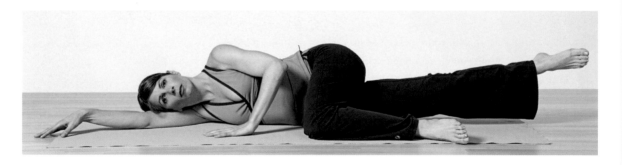

2 Breathe normally as you circle your right leg forward. After five circles, reverse directions.

HEAD TO TOE ALIGNMENT TIPS

❋

1. Try to make a fairly large circle to engage your inner thighs and buttocks.

2. If leg circles are awkward, hold your leg in place.

3. Repeat five leg circles and then reverse directions.

SEAL

This classic Pilates exercise will ease spinal tension after all of your hard work and challenge your balance and control. You can bark like a seal. My students do or they don't get to go home—besides it is fun!

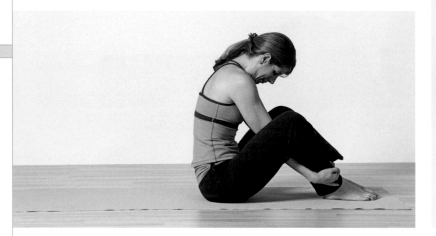

FUSING MIND AND MOTION

✻

Inhale to lift your toes off the ground.

＊＊＊

Exhale to stabilize your pelvis.

＊＊＊

Bark like a seal to have fun!

＊＊＊

Repeat five to eight times.

1. Sit on your bottom with your heels close in, soles of your feet touching the floor. Wrap your arms under your legs reaching under your knees and outside your ankles to grab your feet. Heels are touching.

HEAD TO TOE ALIGNMENT TIPS

✻

1. Clap from your inner thighs, so you engage those muscles.

2. If you are super wobbly, don't clap. Just hold the position.

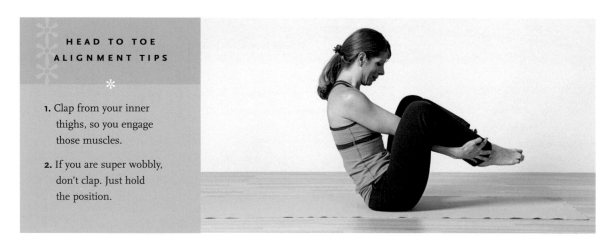

2. Inhale to lift your toes about two to four inches off the floor. Exhale to stabilize your pelvis by scooping your navel to your spine. Breathe normally to clap your heels three times, barking like a seal as you scoop and hug your abs to your spine. Look at your belly the whole time.

STRETCHING YOUR LIMITS

*

Congratulations, you have just completed level two! Although this level includes slightly different exercises than level one, this sequence of exercises will move you closer to the real deal. You now have a working knowledge of the principles of Pilates and should be enjoying some newfound strength. When you feel that you can stable, scoop, and squeeze, then you're ready for Classic Pilates! Here are the chapter highlights:

* * *

In this chapter, you increase the workload for your spine while you increase in strength, balance, mobility, and coordination—all important aspects of functional fitness.

* * *

Functional fitness is a method of training that combines strength, balance, coordination, and stability challenges to prepare your ready for everyday challenges.

* * *

You work with a small hand towel or pillow between your thighs to reinforce the inner pull through the pelvic floor contraction.

* * *

Move with control; absolutely no haphazard movements.

* * *

Concentrate on stabilizing your trunk, scooping your abdominals and now squeezing your inner thighs— stable, scoop, and squeeze.

* * *

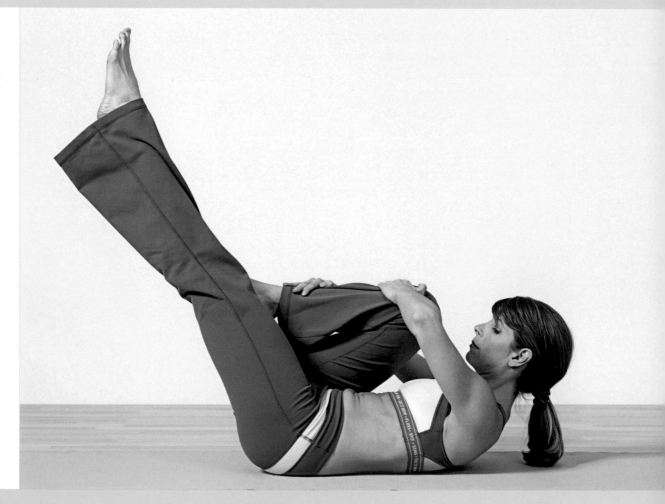

SIMPLY STRIKING

CONGRATULATIONS! This is it—an actual Pilates mat class. These exercises, along with the names and breathing patterns, are the work of Joseph Pilates. And I know you're ready! Although these exercises are slightly different from the earlier chapters, you will see some familiar patterns of movement and, of course, you will recognize the fundamentals. So, let's get your Pilates body moving!

THE PLAN

These exercises are to be done in order because they work your muscles symmetrically. Follow all directions, including the breathing patterns. And don't forget to run through your mental and verbal checklist: head, neck, shoulders, and hips. As the exercises increase in difficulty, you may have a tougher time staying within proper alignment and engaging your mind. Keep at it! Do this workout three to four days a week for as long as you want to stay fit. Here's what you should have gained from level two's workout:

✳ You have eliminated your belly bulging. Well, at least you should be aware of it and have the ability to correct it by either modifying your movement or engaging your deep abdominals.

✳ You have noticeably more muscle tone and strength: You should be enjoying noticeable body results.

✳ You have better posture and stand a little taller.

✳ You have learned how to flow from your center and have a better idea how to initiate movement from your powerhouse.

YOUR GOALS FOR YOUR PILATES WORKOUT

✳ Memorize these mat exercises so you can do them anywhere.

✳ Keep strengthening your powerhouse.

✳ Move with precision and ease of movement.

✳ Gain an "I Like My Body" attitude.

✳ Continue to grow, learn, and move toward having the healthiest body you can.

SEQUENCE OF EXERCISES
LEVEL THREE

✳

PILATES V

THE HUNDRED

ROLL UP

LEG CIRCLES

ROLLING LIKE A BALL

SINGLE LEG STRETCH

DOUBLE LEG STRETCH

SPINE STRETCH

THE SAW

SIDE KICK SERIES
Side Kicks
Heel Beats
Side Passé
Beats on the Belly

SEAL

PILATES V

Up to this point, you have performed modified exercises and have worked within the framework of what is appropriate for your body. You will now fine tune your exercises and work in a Pilates V, meaning the heels of your feet will touch as your toes open about three fingers-width apart—making a "V" with your feet and legs. The Pilates V is important because a slight turn out of your legs will help you engage all of the muscles of your legs between your pelvic floors and inner thigh to your ankles. This V position will also help stabilize your lower body so you can enjoy mega-toning benefits in hard to target areas, such as the butt, hips, and thighs.

HEAD TO TOE ALIGNMENT TIPS

✳

1. This slight turnout happens from your heels and up. If you turn out from your knees only, you may throw off the alignment of your entire leg.

2. Don't turn your feet out too much, for example, as a ballerina would. A wide turnout, which is usually a learned and forced position for dancers, can put too much stress on your knees and ankle joints.

3. If you have a back issue, such as sciatica, stay on the safe side and check with your doctor before turning out. If this is the case, then work with your feet in a parallel position, rather than turning them out, so as not to aggravate your back.

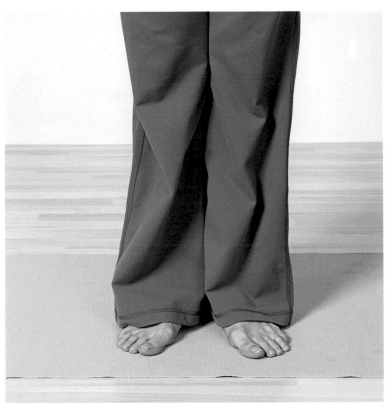

1 In a standing position, put your heels together and open your toes about three fingers apart. Feel the contraction between your inner thighs.

THE HUNDRED

The Hundred will challenge and strengthen your abdominals and breath, warm up your body, increase circulation, and is the first exercise you will do before any other mat exercise. Good form is vital here because if the Hundred is done incorrectly, you may strain your lower back, increase neck and throat tension, and restrict your breathing.

HEAD TO TOE ALIGNMENT TIPS

❋

1. With every exhale, pull your abdominal wall closer to your spine to help stabilize your trunk against the movement of your arms.

2. Your breathing must flow and grow from your core: Inhale through your nose and then prolong your exhale to the point where you feel out of breath.

3. Relax your neck, jaw, and throat.

4. Melt your spine to the mat to help offset your legs lengthening away from your body and the movement of your arms.

5. You can always bend your knees (chapter 5) if you feel the intensity is too great. But try to challenge and strengthen yourself by completing ten breath cycles.

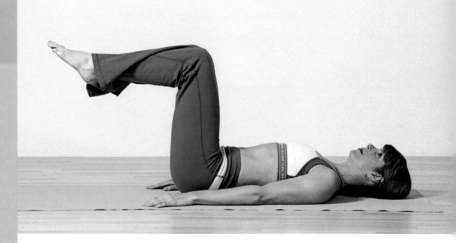

1 Lie on your back with your knees bent and your legs at a 90-degree angle with your feet off the floor. Lengthen your arms by your sides, palms down.

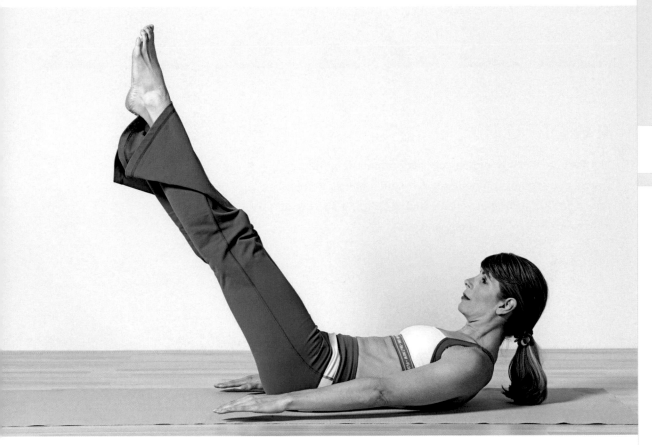

2 In one motion, straighten your legs to the ceiling with your feet in Pilates V. Curl your chin to your chest to lift your shoulders off the floor—neck long. Lift and lengthen your arms past your hips, palms down, and begin pumping your arms by your sides. Fingertips stretch long, wrists are straight, and each pump is about six to eight inches deep—remember to create resistance so your arm muscles work.

FUSING MIND AND MOTION

✳

Inhale for five counts, pumping your arms about six to eight inches.

✳ ✳ ✳

Exhale for five, emptying your lungs as if they are a dirty sponge—squeezing the dirty water (air) out leaves room for the fresh to come in.

✳ ✳ ✳

Complete ten breath cycles, which will add up to the Hundred.

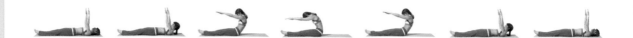

ROLL UP

The Roll Up will strengthen your abdominals, lengthen and stretch your spine, and nourish your spinal bones. Remember, you're peeling your spine off the mat as if lifting a string of pearls—scoop and curl, scoop and curl.

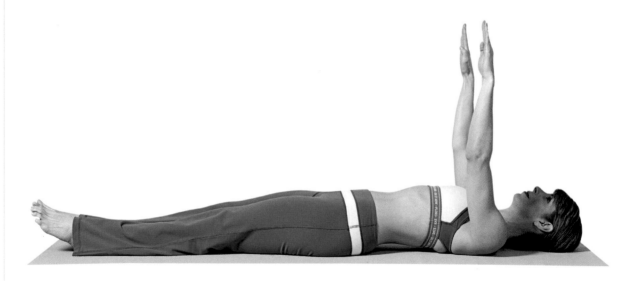

1 Lie on your back with your legs straight, feet in Pilates V. Reach your fingertips to the ceiling. Drop the back of your shoulders against the mat and slide your shoulder blades down your back.

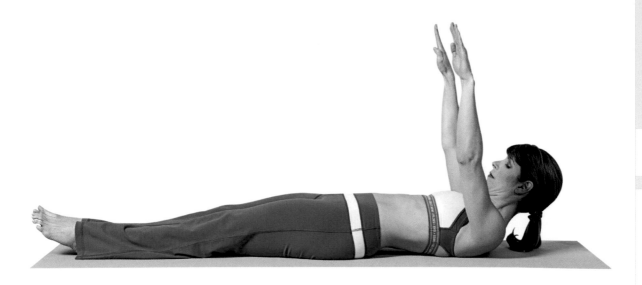

FUSING MIND AND MOTION

*

Inhale to lift your chin to your chest and curl up, peeling your spine off the mat.

***

Exhale to round over, pulling your abdominals to your spine.

***

Inhale to initiate a tilt in your pubic bone.

***

Exhale to scoop and lower each bone of your spine to the mat.

***

You're in motion: don't stop!

***

Repeat three to five times.

2 Inhale to curl your chin to your chest, lifting the back of your shoulders off the mat to look between your arms—keep your neck long.

continued on next page ➤

1. Relax your shoulders. If you let them flow naturally, you'll alleviate upper back tension.

2. Don't jerk or jump as you curl up—smooth, flowing motion is your goal. Likewise, don't plop to the floor. Use your abdominals to control your motion. If you find that you can't control this motion, modify the exercise with the steps in chapter 5.

3. Practice squeezing your inner thighs in the Pilates V. You can always put a small rolled-up hand towel between your legs to encourage this engagement, which will also help control the motion.

4. As you curl up, always gaze at your belly.

5. Don't straighten your spine as you roll up—your spine is rounded. Scoop and curl, scoop and curl.

6. Remember, your neck is an extension of your spine. Don't lift your chin to the ceiling during any phase of the roll up— your spine is curved the whole time.

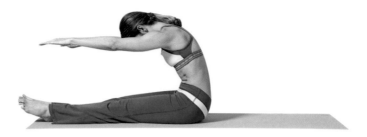

3 Exhale to round over, scooping your navel to your belly at the same time. Your fingers reach long past your toes.

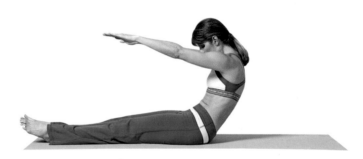

4 Inhale to tilt your pubic bone toward the ceiling, then, as you exhale, roll down so each spinal bone touches the mat. Create length from your pubic bone to the bottom of your breastbone— long and luscious.

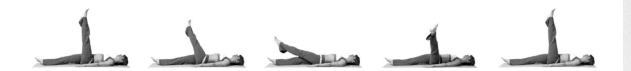

LEG CIRCLES

This exercise will warm up your hips, tighten and tone your hips and thighs, strengthen your abdominals, and nourish your hip joints. At this level, both legs will be straight and the circle will be big. The goal is to challenge your abdominals to keep your hips bones even and your pelvis stable throughout the movement. Imagine your leg circling like a pendulum in your hip socket while your hips remain stable.

1 Lie on your back with your legs extended. Lengthen your arms by your sides, palms down. Neck is long. Move your left knee to your chest and then straighten your leg, toes turned out slightly. While your left leg is active, your right leg presses firmly into the floor—imagine the letter "L." Inhale to lift your toes to your nose.

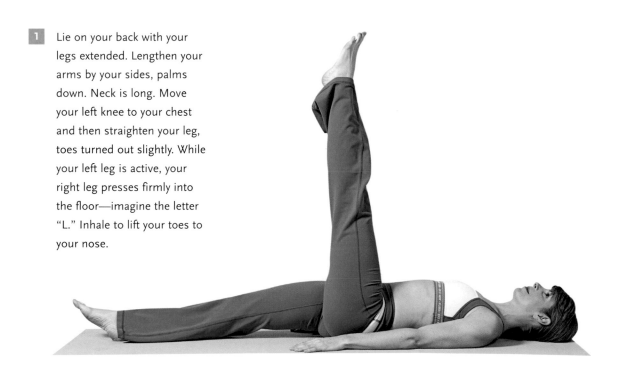

continued on next page ➤

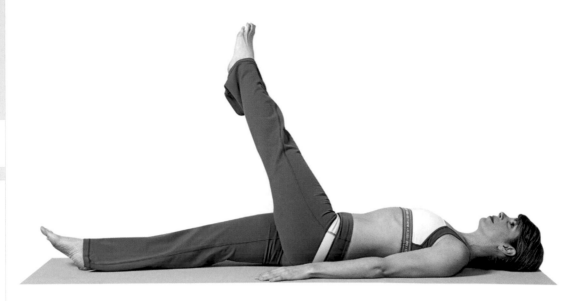

2 Exhale to move your leg across your body, squeezing your inner thighs.

FUSING MIND AND MOTION

✳

Flow your breath with each leg circle.

✳ ✳ ✳

Inhale to lift your toes to your nose.

✳ ✳ ✳

Exhale to draw a circle on the ceiling with your toes: your leg crosses the midline of your body, down to the opposite foot, and circles around to stop at your nose, contracting your inner thighs the whole time.

✳ ✳ ✳

Repeat five leg circles and then reverse the circle for five.

✳ ✳ ✳

Switch legs and repeat.

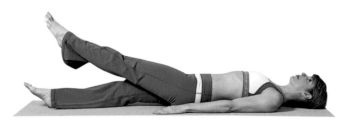

3   Continue to exhale while moving your leg to the opposite foot.

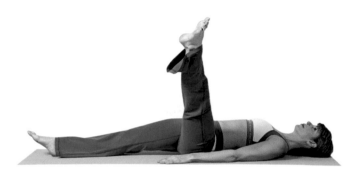

4   Continue to exhale and circle your leg to the side and up toward your nose. Inhale, pause slightly, and then circle your leg again.

**HEAD TO TOE
ALIGNMENT TIPS**

✳

1. Don't rock your hips from side to side as the leg circles. Keep the circles small at first.

2. Stabilize your trunk. If you feel centering is difficult, try pressing the palms of your hands, back of your arms, and the back of your head firmly into the mat to help stabilize your trunk while your leg challenges it.

3. Don't forget to drag out your exhale, which will also assist in pulling your belly button to your spine to help strengthen and stabilize your middle muscles.

4. Imagine a string pulling your big toe to the ceiling to lengthen your leg.

ROLLING LIKE A BALL

This exercise will ease spinal tension, increase spinal flexibility, strengthen and challenge your abdominals and pelvic floors, and increase your balance. This time, your hands are placed in a different, and more advanced, position.

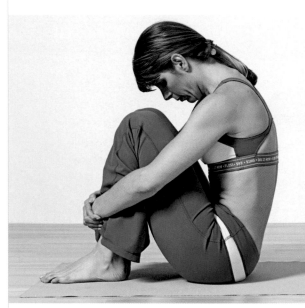

1 Sit at the edge of the mat and slide your heels to your buttocks. Wrap your arms around your legs, elbows out to the sides. Place your hands on your shins, and cross them at the wrists. Your heels stay close to your bottom. Lower your head between your knees so your spine is rounded—lift your belly button up and in.

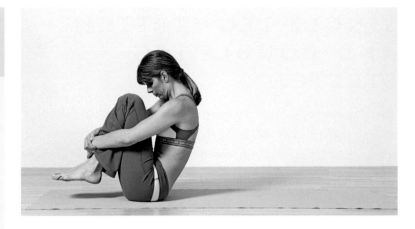

FUSING MIND AND MOTION

✳

Inhale to roll back, squeezing and scooping as you lift your tailbone to the ceiling.

✳✳✳

Exhale to roll up—squeeze, scoop, and stabilize.

2 Lift your toes about two to three inches off the floor. Balance for a second and then inhale to roll back onto your tailbone.

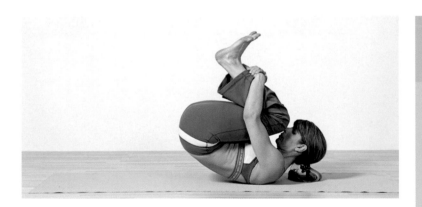

3 Continue to inhale as you roll to the middle portion of your back. Maintain your spinal curve so your head never touches the mat. Stay tight in your ball. Exhale to scoop, roll up, and balance.

HEAD TO TOE ALIGNMENT TIPS

✳

1. Never roll on your neck. Your spine is rounded and your eyes gaze at your belly.

2. Relax your shoulders as they may elevate to your ears, especially if you're struggling to roll up.

3. Flow your breath and motion as if they are one.

4. Squeezing your pelvic floors will give you a little extra boost so you can roll up and balance. So engage those muscles!

SINGLE LEG STRETCH AND DOUBLE LEG STRETCH

These two exercises were designed to transition one into the other without resting. They will build abdominal strength, increase your concentration and focus, improve your coordination, and tone your bottom and thighs. There are many subtle changes—so read the directions carefully.

SINGLE LEG STRETCH

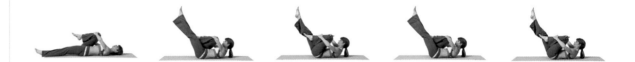

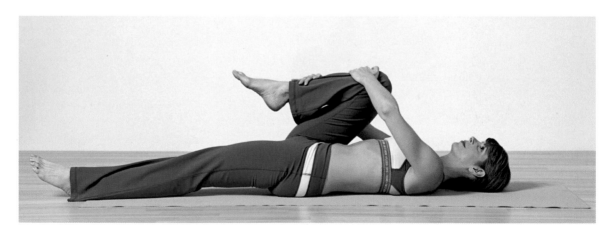

1 Lie on your back with your right knee to your chest. Place your right hand on the outside of your right shin near your ankle and your left hand just below your knee, elbows wide.

FUSING MIND AND MOTION

✳

Inhale gradually, bringing your right knee to your chest with a slight pulse while lengthening your left foot toward the ceiling. Switch legs so your left knee moves toward your chest and your right foot lengthens to the ceiling.

* * *

Exhale gradually, bringing your right knee to your chest with a slight pulse while extending your left foot to the ceiling. Switch legs, so the left knee moves toward your chest and the right foot lengthens to the ceiling—force all the air out of your lungs to flatten your belly. This entire cycle totals one set of leg stretches.

* * *

Repeat four sets.

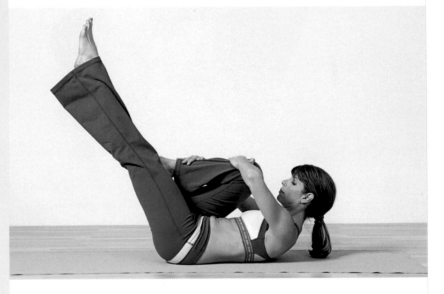

2 In one motion, inhale gradually as you curl your chin to your chest to lift your shoulders off the ground while extending your left leg to the ceiling. Give your right knee two little hugs.

continued on next page ➤

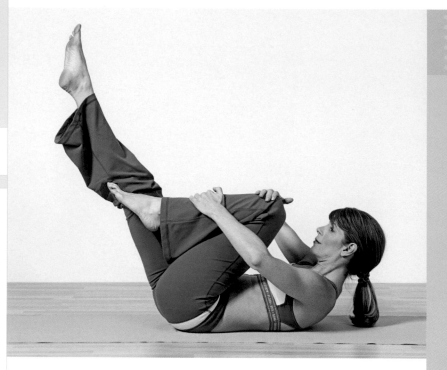

3 Continue to inhale and switch legs so your left leg pulls in and at the same time change your hands so your right hand is on your shin while your left hand is by your knee. Give this leg two hugs, then, as you gradually exhale, switch legs again and hug your right knee for two counts and then your left knee.

HEAD TO TOE ALIGNMENT TIPS

✳

1. Although the hand positioning is mentally challenging, it will keep your knee in alignment with your ankle and hip.

2. Stay strong and stable in your trunk. Don't rock from side to side as the leg moves in and out of positions.

3. As you stretch your legs, lengthen them away from your hips and contract your butt cheeks to tone your bottom and thighs.

4. Motion should flow as you alternate your legs.

5. Keep your head curled up off the floor, lengthening your neck, and quickly move into Double Leg Stretch.

DOUBLE LEG STRETCH

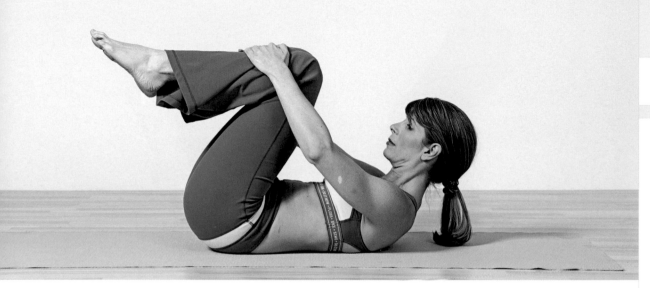

FUSING MIND AND MOTION

✳

Inhale to stretch your arms and legs out.

✳✳✳

Exhale to complete the arm circle while lowering your knees to your chest. Hug your knees to your chest to empty your lungs of air (it's also a nice back stretch).

✳✳✳

Repeat five to eight smooth flowing stretches.

1 Lie on your back with your knees to your chest. While your head is still lifted, wrap your hands around your shins. Give your knees a little hug to exhale the air from your lungs.

continued on next page ➤

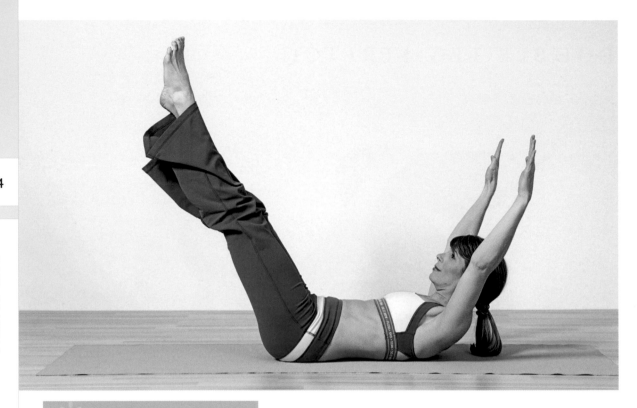

1. If your neck tires before your body, check your head placement. Your neck is long as you gaze between your thighs. If the problem still persists, your abdominals might not be strong enough yet. You can rest between these two exercises if needed or review the steps in chapter 5. But please don't stress your neck.

2. Stabilize your trunk against the movement. There should not be any trunk movement while your limbs are challenging and strengthening your abdominals.

3. Don't let your head drop to the floor or lift your chin to the ceiling as the arms circle behind. Gaze at your toes.

2 Inhale to lengthen your legs to a slight angle so your toes reach long toward the ceiling while reaching your arms over your head. Circle your arms behind you and around. Imagine that your toes are pulled in one direction while your fingers stretch in the other direction, both secured by a solid and stable torso. Exhale to finish the arm circle while pulling your knees to your chest, giving your knees a hug with your hands. Your tailbone should remain on the floor and your pelvis is stable—scoop your navel to your spine.

SPINE STRETCH

Spine Stretch will ease your spinal tension, put a little space between each spinal bone, nourish the spinal column, and reinforce the stacking of each bone of your spine while you're in a seated position.

FUSING MIND AND MOTION

❋

Inhale to prepare, focusing on perfect posture: your shoulders over your hips while your shoulder blades slide down your back. Ground your butt bones into the floor while stacking all of the bones of your spine directly on top of one another.

✱✱✱

Exhale forcibly to reach your fingertips past your toes while rounding your spine so you gaze at your belly.

✱✱✱

Repeat three to five stretches.

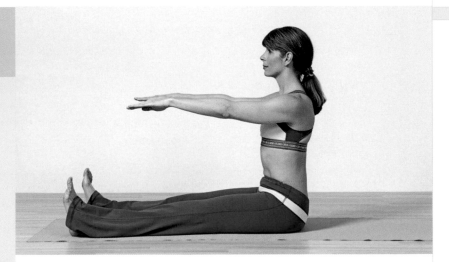

1 Sit on the mat with your legs extended a little wider than shoulder-width apart, feet flexed. Lift your arms so they are parallel to your legs. Navel is pulled up and in under your ribs. Inhale to grow tall from within.

continued on next page ➤

1. Sit up out of your hips and visualize your head floating to the clouds. Use your inner thighs, bottom, and belly to help create a stable and straight spine out from the top of your head.

2. Cement your legs and bottom to the mat as your round over—absolutely no movement in the lower half of your body.

3. You're making the letter "C" with your spine, rather than straightening it. Although you might feel your hamstrings stretch, the goal of this exercise is to round your spine to stretch it.

4. This exercise focuses on postural awareness. Maintaining a neutral spine is important to the health of your spinal bones. No slumping in your lower back!

5. If you can't sit up out of your hips, place a small pad under your bottom or bend your knees as you see in the modified picture.

6. If you feel any pressure in the back of your knees, bend them slightly. They should not be locked, pushing down into the floor.

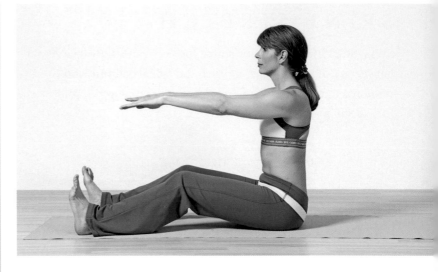

2 To modify this exercise, bend your knees or put a small pad under your bottom.

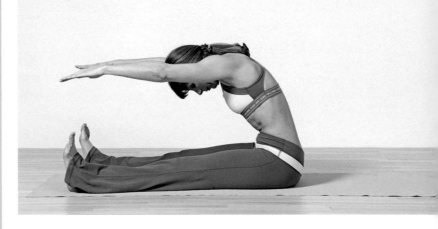

3 Exhale to round over, dropping your chin to your chest while gazing at your belly. Even though your fingertips are reaching past your toes, pull your navel up toward the ceiling to stretch your spine. Imagine a porcupine with sharp needles under your belly—this should get you to scoop your navel to your spine a little deeper. Inhale to roll up and re-stack your spine, bone by bone.

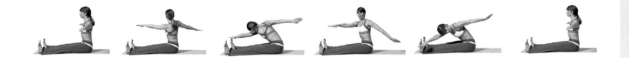

THE SAW

The Saw will strengthen your oblique abdominals, cleanse your lungs of all its impurities, and is the ultimate waist trimmer.

FUSING MIND AND MOTION

✳

Inhale to grow tall from within and stack your spinal bones.

✳✳✳

Exhale to twist in the movement: one, two, three pulses to twist a little farther, blowing out every ounce of air.

✳✳✳

Repeat three to five times.

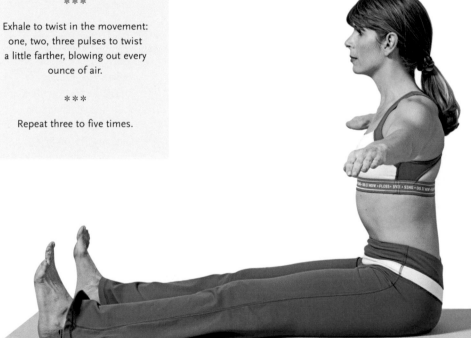

1 Sit tall on the mat with your legs extended a little wider than shoulder-width apart, feet flexed. Lift your arms out to the sides of your body and reach your fingertips long, palms down.

continued on next page ➤

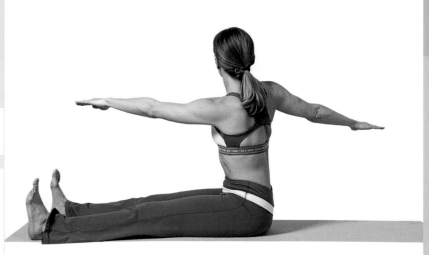

2 Inhale to grow tall within, lifting your ribs slightly up, then begin to twist, initiating the movement from your waist. A twist should never come from your lower spinal bones, because they don't rotate.

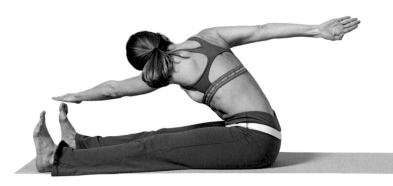

3 Exhale to reach your left hand to your right foot and past the pinky toe. Imagine your left pinky finger "sawing" off your right pinky toe while your left ear moves closer to your right knee. With each pulse, twist a little farther, exhaling every ounce of air out of your lungs. Inhale to return to the starting position.

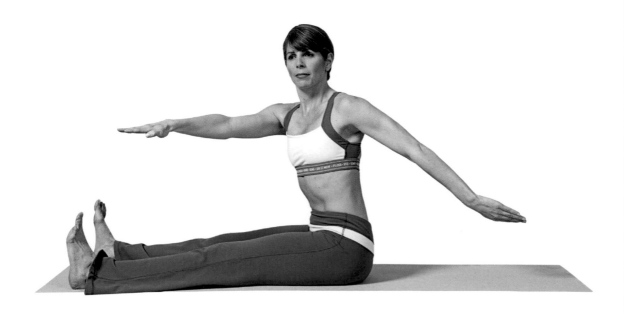

4 Inhale to grow tall within, lifting your ribs slightly up, then twist your right hand to your left foot—your ribs initiate the twist.

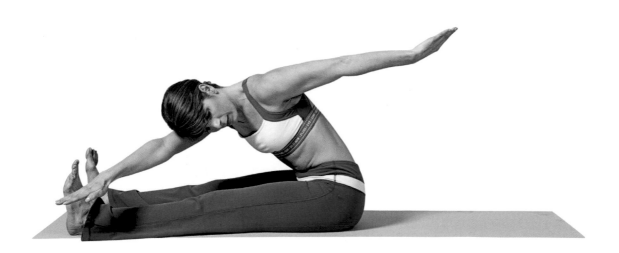

5 Exhale to reach your right hand to your left foot and past the pinky toe; move your right ear closer to your left knee as you pulse for three counts while stretching your right hand behind you, palm up. With each pulse, twist a little farther, exhaling every ounce of air out of your lungs. Inhale to return to the starting position.

SIDE KICK SERIES

✳

SIDE KICKS

This leg exercise will tone and tighten your thighs and buttocks, challenge your trunk stability and balance in an advanced side-lying position, and open and stretch tight hips and hamstrings.

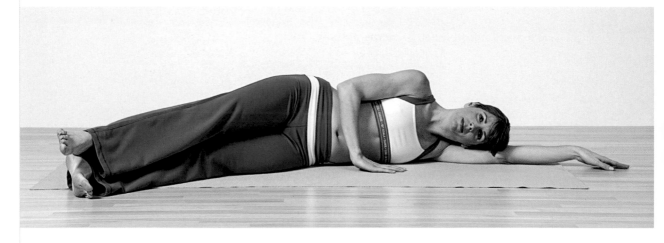

1 Lie on your right side with your legs extended, both hip bones stacked on top of one another. Your feet are in a Pilates V. Straighten your right arm and rest your head on it and then place your left arm so your palm is down on the mat in front of your torso; relax your shoulders. Lift both legs at the same time and lower them in front of your body to about a 45-degree angle—your body will make the shape of a banana. You'll perform the entire leg series on your right side and then transition to the left side to complete your leg work.

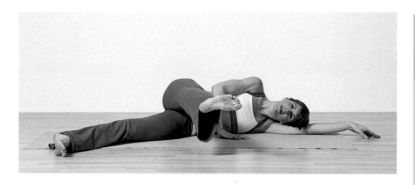

2 Lift the top leg to hip-height. Inhale to swing your leg forward with a double kick: swing your leg forward and then quickly add a smaller kick or pulse. The top leg is directly hip-height and parallel to the floor—you might feel a slight hamstring stretch. Make sure your hips stay stacked on top of one another and maintain a neutral pelvis.

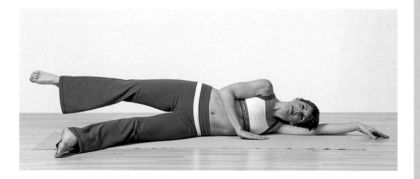

3 Exhale to swing your leg back with a double kick—swinging the leg back and then quickly adding another small kick or pulse to engage your bottom. As your leg swings back, you will challenge your trunk stability and tone your butt!

HEAD TO TOE ALIGNMENT TIPS

✳

1. When you set your body in position for these exercises, proper alignment is critical—keep your hips square, shoulders relaxed away from your ears, your center solid, and your supporting elbow lifted to the ceiling and close to the body to keep you stable.

2. As your leg swings forward, its weight may roll the hip forward as well. Remember, your hips should remain even and stacked on top of one another.

3. As your leg swings back, its weight may cause you to lift your ribs and arch your lower back. Pull you navel to your spine by focusing on your rib-to-hip connection—you need to challenge and engage all your abdominal muscles.

4. Relax your head, neck, and shoulders. Watch for needless tension in your upper back.

5. Stay solid in your core. Even though your legs are moving to challenge your center, it must remain stable and engaged.

6. After five to ten sets, return to the starting position to move into the next exercise, Heel Beats.

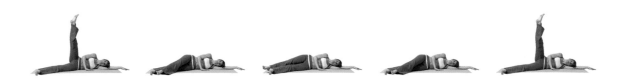

HEEL BEATS

This leg exercise will tone and tighten your buttocks and thighs, especially your inner thighs; challenge your trunk stability and balance in an advanced side lying position; open and stretch tight hips; and encourage you to contract your pelvic floor muscles.

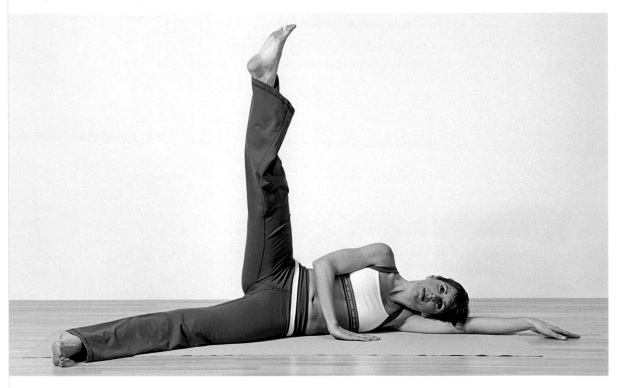

1 Lie on your left side with your legs extended, making sure both hip bones are stacked on top of one another. Your feet are in a Pilates V. Extend your left arm out on the floor and place your right arm in front of you with your palm on the mat in front of your torso; relax your shoulders. Lift both legs at the same time and lower them to the ground in front of your body to about a 45-degree angle—your body makes the shape of a banana. Inhale to lift the right leg to the ceiling. Your knee faces up as your toes lengthen—imagine miles and miles of leg.

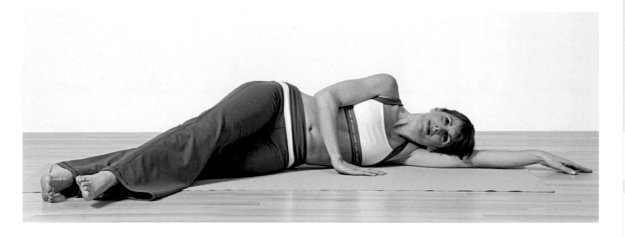

2 Exhale to lower your right leg to just above the floor, leading with your heel and contracting between your thighs. As your leg nears the floor, lengthen your leg and quickly pulse your heel in front of your toes.

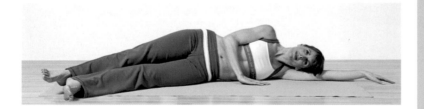

3 Continue exhaling as you quickly pulse your right heel behind your left heel. Then, as you inhale, lift your right leg up to the ceiling again.

HEAD TO TOE ALIGNMENT TIPS

*

1. Sometimes your hips will tend to sink back to the mat as your leg lifts or your chest and hips will collapse toward one another. Remain lifted and stable in your center with your hips stacked on top of one another.

2. As your top leg lowers to your bottom leg, lengthen it longer than your bottom heel.

3. Relax your head, neck, and shoulders.

4. Again, nothing moves except for your kicking leg.

3. Repeat five to ten times then move directly into Side Passé, staying on the same side.

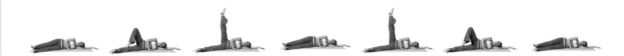

SIDE PASSÉ

This leg exercise will tone and tighten your buttocks, thighs, and pelvic floors; challenge your trunk stability and balance in an advanced side lying position; open and stretch tight hips; and nourish your hip joints.

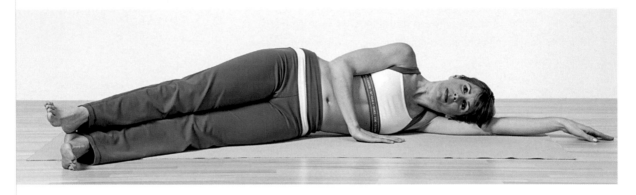

1 Lie on your left side with your legs extended, making sure both hip bones are stacked on top of one another. Your feet are in a Pilates V. Extend your left arm out on the floor and place your right arm, palm down, in front of your torso; relax your shoulders. Lift both legs at the same time and lower them in front of your body to about a 45 degree angle—your body makes the shape of a banana.

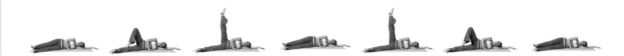

HEAD TO TOE ALIGNMENT TIPS

✳

1. Again, your hips will have a tendency to sink back to the mat as your leg lifts or your chest and hips will collapse toward one another. Lift your leg only as high as you can maintain your alignment. Remain lifted and stable in your center. Your hips are stable and stacked on top of one another.

2. As your top leg lowers, engage your pelvic floors and inner thighs to get maximum toning benefits.

3. Relax your head, neck, and shoulders.

4. Sometimes, hip tightness can prevent you from lifting your knee to the ceiling. Do what you can, but know that lifting your knee to the ceiling opens and stretches your hips; this is your ultimate goal.

5. Repeat three times and then reverse the direction of the passé: your leg moves straight up, bends down, and then slides along the bottom leg for three more.

6. Transition to Beats on the Belly, staying on the same side. After completing Beats on the Belly, you will switch sides to do the Side Kick Series on your other side.

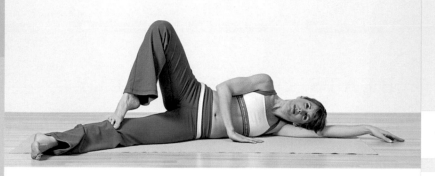

2   Inhale to bend your right leg and slide your toes along the inside of your left leg so your knee lifts to the ceiling.

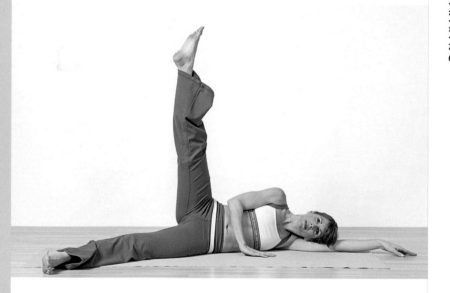

3   Continue inhaling to straighten your leg to the ceiling, toes lengthening long. Exhale to lower your right leg so it's even with your left leg, extending the top heel past your bottom foot.

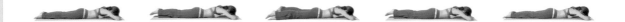

BEATS ON THE BELLY

This leg exercise will tone and tighten your thighs and buttocks and challenge the muscles of your back.

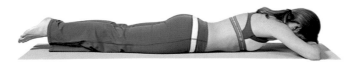

1 Roll on your belly and lengthen your legs long from your center. Place your hands over your head and cross them at the wrists, so your elbows are out to the sides. Rest your head on your forearms. As always, give your back a little support by lifting your belly button to your spine.

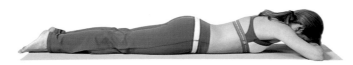

2 Lift your legs about two to three inches off the mat.

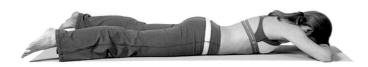

3 Inhale as you click and beat your heels together, counting to five. Exhale and continue to beat your heels together for another set of five, for a total of ten counts.

HEAD TO TOE ALIGNMENT TIPS

❋

1. Again, pick the pit of your belly up toward your spine while relaxing your back. Remember, this action is not a forced lift, but a gentle one with support for your low back.

2. Watch and feel for strain in your lumbar spine. This lift comes from your bottom, so engage your buttocks!

3. Relax your shoulders, neck, and upper back.

4. Your legs are working to strengthen and tone your inner thighs and butt while your center provides stability and support.

5. Rest in Child's Pose for a few minutes. Then do the Side Kick Series on the other leg.

SEAL

The Seal is your grand finale! This time, you will roll and clap at the same time. This exercise will cool you down and relieve any spinal tension, but balance and control are still vital to making this exercise work.

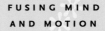

FUSING MIND AND MOTION

*

Inhale to prepare for the movement; drop your chin to your chest.

***

Exhale to roll back.

***

Inhale to roll up, then clap your heels together three times.

***

Repeat eight to ten times.

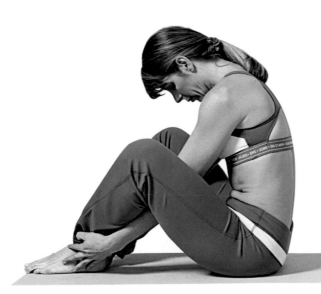

1 Sit at the edge of your mat and slide your heels to your buttocks. Wrap your arms under your legs and around to place your hands on the outside of your ankles. Gaze at your belly as you scoop your navel and you curl your chin to your chest, maintaining a rounded spine.

continued on next page ➤

HEAD TO TOE ALIGNMENT TIPS

✳

1. When you clap, try to engage your inner thighs as well.

2. Never roll onto your neck; it's the upper back and shoulders that absorb the weight of your body. I like to say, "Give your butt up to the Heavens."

3. Don't forget to bark like a seal; it's a fun way to finish up!

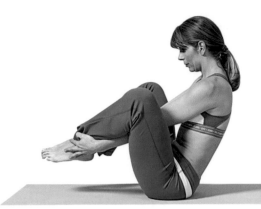

2 Inhale to lift your feet off the floor and scoop and stabilize to clap your heels together. Feel free to bark like a seal—it's fun!

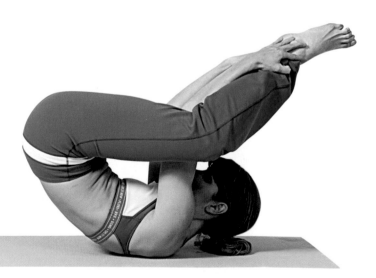

3 Exhale to roll back and lift your butt in the air, shifting your body weight to your upper back. Your head should never touch the floor. Inhale and roll up scooping your belly, finding your balance to clap your heels together again.

STRETCHING YOUR LIMITS

✳

That's a wrap! As you approach the end of this workout, I hope you feel mentally and physically engaged and have stretched your limits.

* * *

Gain an "I Like My Body" attitude!

* * *

Continue to grow, learn, and move toward having the healthiest body you can.

* * *

ACKNOWLEDGMENTS

IT TAKES A VILLAGE TO PUBLISH A BOOK AND
I'm blessed to have had a wonderful team at Fair Winds Press (a
division of Rockport Publishers)! Thank you so much Holly
Schmidt for believing in this project and Ken Fund for signing off
on it. This book wouldn't even be a book if it weren't for the
women of Gilda's Club North Texas. Every time I teach them,
those women teach me and leave me inspired to do more, laugh
more, and live life to its fullest; I'm indebted for such a gift.

I'm pretty sure that I have the best editor in publishing, Donna
Raskin. I'm especially grateful for your support and your smarts.
Special thanks to Rhiannon Soucy for making my stay in
Gloucester a memorable one; Brigid Carroll, who tweaked my
manuscript in its earliest stages; and Kristna Evans, my copyedi-
tor, who put her finishing touches on it. On the brilliant creative
team, I am so lucky to have people like Silke Braun! Thank you
once again for your vision as to what this book should look like
and to Claire MacMaster for making it happen. Allan Penn, you

are a brilliant photographer and I'm in awe of your expertise. Thank you and your assistant, Bevan—you are too cute for making sure each detail was perfect—right down to my feet! I'm also grateful to Deborah Coull, who is an old soul, and Lesley Griffin from the Deborah Coull Salon for doing my hair and makeup—gosh, I wish I had their skills! A special thank you to Lululemon Athletica for providing the most gorgeous clothing for my photo shoot.

Thank you to my family. Even though, we're spread across the nation, we talk everyday. I'm especially indebted to Kjehl Rasmussen for all of your emotional support and career guidance. And then there is my long time writing coach, Janet Harris, who gives her prose blessing to each of my writing projects. Of course, I'm grateful that I had incredible instructors, such as Karen Sanzo PT, and Colleen Glenn, to learn Pilates from. And finally, a special thanks to my students, whom I continue to learn from everyday!

ABOUT THE AUTHOR

KARON KARTER IS A FITNESS EXPERT who writes regularly for the *Dallas Morning News* and various magazines. She has also written several books, including *The Complete Idiot's Guide to the Pilates Method, The Core Strength Workout,* and T*he Complete Idiot's Guide to Body Ball Fitness.*

Karter has worked for Dr. Kenneth Cooper's Institute for Aerobic Research supervising new corporate health programs, such as Dow Chemical's "Up with Life" and Texas Instruments' "Life Track" program. She has received several certifications, including the Aerobics Institute's Physical Fitness Specialist Course and Group Leadership Course. She is a certified and classically trained Pilates instructor and currently teaches the methods of Joseph Pilates in her home town of Dallas, Texas.

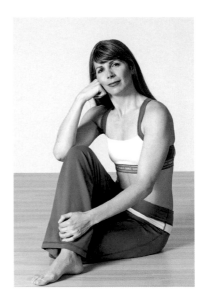

Also Available from Fair Winds Press

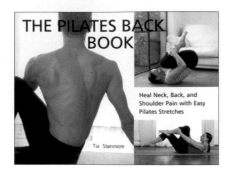

THE PILATES BACK BOOK
by Tia Stanmore
ISBN: 1-931412-89-8
$17.95
Paperback; 128 pages
Available wherever books are sold

HEAL NECK, BACK, AND SHOULDER PAIN WITH EASY PILATES STRETCHES
Most of us will experience back pain at some point in our lives, often as a result of injury or poor posture. By building inner muscular strength and flexibility, this Pilates-based exercise program gives real and lasting benefits for people suffering from back ache, a sore neck or strained muscles. It can prevent you from experiencing injuries and postural problems and help you recover more quickly if you do.

The step-by-step exercises are easy to follow whether you are familiar with Pilates or a newcomer. If you need to concentrate on a specific area of your back the Upper Torso and the Lumbo-pelvic programs will guide you through the exercises most beneficial to you.

Tia Stanmore is a member of the Pilates Foundation and is a Pilates instructor at The Third Space in London. She has presented numerous conferences and training sessions on the use of Pilates in Physiotherapy. She is a Board Member for the Dance UK Physiotherapy Advisory Board and has developed a role in injury prevention and in skill training for dancers.

Also Available from Fair Winds Press

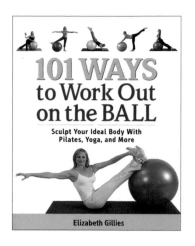

101 WAYS TO WORK OUT ON THE BALL
by Elizabeth Gillies
ISBN: 1-59233-084-3
$19.95 (£12.99)
Paperback; 176 pages
Available wherever books are sold

SCULPT YOUR IDEAL BODY WITH PILATES, YOGA, AND MORE
Everyone loves the workout ball! It can help with weight training, Pilates, yoga, and even cardio and stretching moves. And nobody knows the ball like Liz Gillies. *101 Ways to Work Out on the Ball* gives you exercises that will strengthen, lengthen, tone, and stretch your body like no other form of exercise can. The moves will work for beginners, intermediate, and advanced exercisers; some even require weights to sculpt your arms and legs while strengthening your core. The program includes workout plans and tips for progressing through the series.

Liz Gillies develops and stars in numerous videos including *Zone Pilates*, *Stability Ball Workouts*, *Stability Ball for Dummies*, and most recently her own "Core Fitness" line of videos. She is the owner and artistic director of The Insidescoop Studio in New York, where she has been certifying teachers in the Pilates Method since 1997. She is regularly featured in news programs and national publications.

Also Available from Fair Winds Press

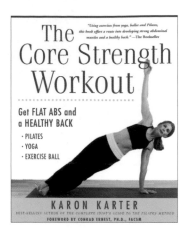

THE CORE STRENGTH WORKOUT
by Karon Karter
ISBN: 1-59233-057-6
$19.95
Paperback; 208 pages

GET FIT TO THE CORE!
Transform your body with the exercises dancers, gymnasts, and Olympic athletes count on to stay strong, slim, and sexy. With *The Core Strength Workout* as your guide, you'll target the critical torso muscles that make the difference between fat and fabulous. You'll walk taller, sleeker, and leaner within weeks!

No matter what your current level of fitness, you'll find easy and effective routines that work for you. Inside these beautiful full-color pages, celebrated fitness instructor and author Karon Karter shows you how to:

• Flatten your tummy with Pilates and yoga moves
• Strengthen your back and improve your posture
• Use the exercise ball to tighten your torso
• Progress from beginner to intermediate to advanced routines
• Work your abs in only ten minutes

Tap into the fitness trend of the decade with *The Core Strength Workout*. You—and your torso—will be glad you did!

Karon is the author of *The Healthy Flier*, *The Complete Idiot's Guide to Kickboxing* and *The Complete Idiot's Guide to the Pilates Method*. She writes for *The Dallas Morning News* and *D Magazine*, specializing in fitness, health and travel topics. She currently teaches Pilates and a variety of other fitness classes in Dallas, Texas.